SIRTFOOD DIET

2 BOOKS IN 1:
SIRTFOOD DIET PLAN AND COOKBOOK

THE MOST COMPLETE GUIDE TO ACTIVATE YOUR
SKINNY GENE, BURN FAT AND LOSE WEIGHT.
INCLUDES DELICIOUS RECIPES AND AN
EXCLUSIVE MEAL PLAN

Isabel Taylor

COPYRIGHT

TABLE OF CONTENTS

SIRTFOOD DIET PLAN

LOSE 7 LBS IN 7 DAYS.

THE NUTRITION GUIDE WITH AN EXCLUSIVE MEAL PLAN TO LOSE WEIGHT FAST, BURN FAT AND PREVENT CANCER. DISCOVER THE POWER OF SUPERFOODS AND CHANGE YOUR LIFE

Isabel Taylor

INTRODUCTION

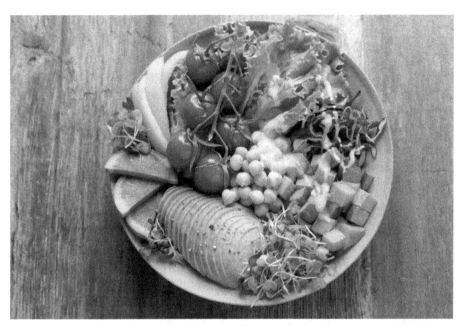

Much the same as Keto and Whole30, the Sirtfood Diet often radicalizes how you regularly eat by requesting that you hold back on dinners. While all diets often hold fast to some type of a calorie-limit, Caldwell says it's critical to consider your own lifestyle and consider what you need for the duration of the day. "Actually, there is nothing supernatural about sirtfoods specifically — being rich in polyphenols, they do have calming properties, yet the exploration doesn't bolster them having any additional adequacy for weight loss."

If you're hell bent on checking out the Sirtfood Diet, first investigation by joining a greater amount of the diet's mark staples into what you're as of now eating at home. "Consolidating polyphenol-rich nourishments, including those on the sirtfood list, can be useful in forestalling or diminishing fiery sicknesses like cardiovascular malady," she prompts. "Avoid the underlying prohibitive advances and recommended green juices, and rather choose including cell reinforcement rich nourishments to your eating design in a manner you appreciate."

If the diet's rundown of commended fixings appears to be somewhat inadequate with regards to, you're not the only one — numerous wellbeing specialists condemn the Sirtfood Diet for being exceptionally prohibitive. Beckerman says she has never prescribed the Sirtfood Diet to any of her customers as a result of its tight calorie limitations. "While I praise the Sirtfood Diet for advancing the utilization of genuine fixings, I censure it for its advancement of calorie limitation and undesirable eating rules." Like numerous different diets that expel nutrition classes from normal utilization, Beckerman says the Sirtfood Diet may surely prompt "disarranged eating" as it additionally mixes components from discontinuous fasting plans in with the general mish-mash.

McKenzie Caldwell, MPH, RDN, who represents considerable authority in ladies' nourishment and pregnancy dietary wellbeing specifically, says that the carbohydrate levels related with the diet are by a wide margin it's most exceedingly awful quality. "1,000 calories for every day is suitable for a youngster between the ages of 2 and 4," she says, referring to current dietary rules conveyed by the Mayo Clinic. "Not exclusively is this insufficient vitality to help a grown-up body, it is absurd to expect to fit in all the large scale and micronutrients a grown-up needs in that measure of nourishment... The diet may cause weight loss in the present moment just as a result of its caloric limitation."

Above all, in any case, both nourishment specialists concur that there is practically no clinical proof to help this diet being sound for continued weight loss. "There is positively no proof to back up any cases that the Sirtfood Diet beneficially affects solid weight loss," Beckerman says. "The makers of the diet guarantee to have put members at their own exercise center on the diet, however this narrative guessed study has not been distributed nor approved by obvious specialists or researchers."

WHAT IS SIRTFOOD?

Of late, Adele has been standing out as truly newsworthy past her dazzling voice: After venturing out looking slimmer than expected, a free for all of reports guarantee that the 31-year-old "Somebody Like You" artist shed pounds by following the Sirtfood Diet, a calorie-limiting eating plan, after her separation with her significant other Simon Konecki.

This isn't the first run through Adele's name has been related with the Sirtfood Diet. In 2016, the New York Post guaranteed the artist shed 30 pounds by eating nourishments rich in sirtuins, a.k.a. proteins that can be found in specific nourishments (they likewise happen normally in the body). Her previous Pilates teacher Camila Goodis additionally disclosed to The Sun that she accepted the star's weight loss was "90%" diet.

Adele hasn't freely remarked on the gossipy tidbits twirling around her figure (for what reason ought to she?!), yet her coach Pete Geracimo (who additionally works with Pippa Middleton) evidently prefers to put his customers on the Sirtfood Diet.

Also, as the seventh most Googled diet in 2019, individuals obviously need to realize what it's about. Here, dietitians and a specialist clarify what the Sirtfood Diet involves, the nourishments it empowers, and whether it's a genuine method to get in shape long haul.

What is the Sirtfood Diet?

The Sirtfood Diet depends on the book by a similar name that was composed by Aidan Goggins and Glen Matten. The diet centers around eating supposed sirtfoods, a gathering of "wonderfoods" that incorporate supplement rich choices like kale, cocoa, strawberries, and espresso.

The Sirtfood Diet

The thought is that sure nourishments actuate sirtuins in your body (a sort of protein found in plants) that supposedly gloat a large number of advantages, such as shielding cells from irritation, launching your digestion, turning around maturing, and initiating your "thin quality pathways," according to the diet's site.

Some exploration, similar to one 2018 survey distributed in the diary Circulation Research, proposes that sirtuins may help forestall age-related decrease (in mice, in any event). Another survey distributed in Frontiers in Endocrinology reasons that sirtuins may help forestall insulin obstruction and interminable aggravation. In any case, once more, this depended on creature examines.

While sirtuins are viewed as sound, there's still a ton people don't think about them. "The exploration on sirtuins is promising yet more is unquestionably required, particularly on people, to decide whether any of the cases can be definitively validated," says Keri Gans, M.S., R.D.N., C.D.N., a sustenance specialist situated in New York City.

The Sirtfood Diet just notices a couple sirtfoods on its site and blog, yet these choices make the cut, which are all supplement thick and beneficial to eat normally:

- green tea
- cocoa powder
- turmeric
- kale
- onions
- parsley
- broccoli
- cauliflower
- olive oil
- olives
- apples
- red grapes

- chocolate
- slick fish, similar to salmon, trout, and mackerel

What does the Sirtfood Diet dinner plan resemble?

The diet is separated into two stages, and devotees are urged to do them whenever they have a feeling that they need a weight loss help.

- Stage one:

This goes on for seven days and it's additionally separated. During the initial three days, you'll have three sirtfood green juices and one normal dinner that is rich in sirtfoods—for an aggregate of 1,000 calories every day. On days four through seven, you'll have two green juices and two day by day dinners for a sum of 1,500 calories every day.

- Stage two:

This is a 14-day "upkeep stage" that is intended to assist you with getting in shape at a relentless pace. During this stage, you'll eat three adjusted suppers that are rich in sirtfoods, alongside one green juice. It's indistinct whether this stage has a set calorie admission.

The juices for the most part comprise of matcha, the herb lovage, and buckwheat. Concerning the dinners, plans incorporate soy yogurt with berries, pecans, and dim chocolate, an omelet with bacon, red chicory, and parsley, a pita with turkey, cheddar, and hummus, and sautéed prawns with kale and buckwheat noodles.

When you're finished with the stages, you should take a gander at the Sirtfood Diet as a lifestyle. "You are empowered, when you've finished the initial three weeks, to keep eating a diet rich in sirtfoods and to keep drinking your day by day green squeeze," the diet's site says.

The official site additionally prescribes that you quit working out or decreasing your standard daily practice during the main stage, since you're not taking in numerous calories. Be that as it may, when the diet turns into a lifestyle for you, it supports working out (and eating protein an hour after you work out to fix muscles and decrease irritation).

Can the Sirtfood Diet assist you with shedding pounds?

Truly, you'll likely get in shape on the diet. "A great many people unquestionably will get in shape during stage one, since they are most likely expending way less calories than they normally do," says Gans. While a ton of this might be water weight, it's conceivable to lose real muscle versus fat as well.

In any case, that doesn't mean it's solid. "It appears to be gimmicky," says Jessica Cording, M.S., R.D., writer of The Little Book of Game-Changers. "Any diet where there's a cycle of excessively prohibitive eating and support isn't generally practical."

What are the drawbacks of the Sirtfood Diet?

To begin with, stage one of the diet is "somewhat extraordinary," says Scott Keatley, R.D., of Keatley Medical Nutrition Therapy. "A 1,000 calorie-diet is beneath what is utilized in practically all human research considers since it is regarded dangerous." People can lose liquid and slender bulk while having a caloric admission this low, and it can disturb your digestion, he says.

Limiting your caloric admission this intensely must be "alright" for a couple of days, however it's truly not perfect, says weight loss master Michael Russo, M.D., a bariatric specialist at MemorialCare Surgical Weight Loss Center at Orange Coast Medical Center in Fountain Valley, CA. "It's extremely imperative to focus on what sorts of calories that is no joke," he says. "Getting sufficient protein is urgent, in light of the fact that they're the structure squares of the body."

The squeezing part isn't actually a hit with specialists, either. "I'm not an enormous fanatic of making juice out of nourishments, particularly when we're talking weight loss, as the blender is doing a ton of the work your body ought to do," Keatley says. Green juice is often a lot of lower in gut-filling fiber than you'd get if you just ate the fixings themselves, Cording says, which will undoubtedly leave you hungry.

The diet is additionally inadequate with regards to an instructive part of helping individuals better comprehend what nourishments are useful for their wellbeing, and how to create good dieting examples because of how prohibitive it is, Cording includes. At long last, there are actually no rules past the two stages—except if you purchase the Sirtfood Diet books.

Main concern: If you would like to attempt the Sirtfood Diet, be practical about your desires.

You ought to likewise talk with a dietitian or specialist before your drastically diminish your calorie allow and glug a huge amount of juice for the sake of weight loss.

Eventually, the Sirtfood Diet isn't supported by significant research, so you're likely happier after a solid diet you realize you can adhere to reliably (or an all the more scientifically-demonstrated choice, similar to the Mediterranean diet), practicing normally, and getting a lot of rest.

WHAT YOU NEED TO KNOW ABOUT SIRTFOOD DIET PLAN

While Adele never neglects to dazzle millions with her beautiful voice, her ongoing occasion pictures have people talking! Gazing slimmer and conditioned upward than before, the 31-year-old's change is one to look for inspiration from!

All things considered, imagine a scenario in which we let you know, the accomplishment behind Adele's change is eating brilliant. A fanatic of 'sirtfood diet', Adele followed this diet to get thinner and get into a more advantageous and (obviously, great) shape.

What is the sirtfood diet?

The most recent diet rinse which has the world raving about it follows a scientific way to deal with fight weight gain.

The diet advances on the utilization of 'sirtfoods', which are some uncommon nourishments which work by enacting certain protein chains in the body, known as sirtuins. According to science, these cancer prevention agent operators go about as protectants that help hinder maturing, support digestion and control the body's irritation, thus helping in fat loss.

Studies have likewise discovered that the sirtfood diet can assist individuals with losing as much as seven pounds (3 kilos) in less than seven days' time.

As mind boggling and scientific as this diet plan sounds, the diet urges you to incorporate probably the most normally discovered kitchen fixings just as some liberal nourishments. Some normal nourishments permitted right now food sources like oranges, dim chocolates, parsley, turmeric, kale, and even red wine.

The diet, however viewed as a craze, focusses on keeping up a prohibitive weight loss methodology multi week. While the initial three days makes you limit your calorie admission to 1000kcal (expending three sirt nourishment green squeezes and having a dinner). The rest of the days, you are permitted to expand your calorie admission to 1500kcal and have two suppers per day (alongside two sirtfood juices). Post this, the support stage prescribes you to eat up to three adjusted nourishments rich in sirtuin, combined with a successful workout methodology to get thinner, making it even more maintainable.

Since it is fairly prohibitive in nature, many remain careful about the diet plan working over the long haul. The diet confines your calorie allow and can void you of other required supplements, in this way, it's anything but a long haul, economical diet plan for weight loss.

Adele has likewise decreased her eating propensities and watches her carbs. Sharing some more privileged insights, Adele additionally said that she has removed tea and sugar from her diet, something which she wanted to have! In a meeting, she stated,

"I used to cry however now I sweat. I used to drink ten cups [of tea] a day with two sugars in each so I was on 20 sugars per day. Presently I don't drink tea any longer and I have more vitality than any other time in recent memory."

Wellness privileged insights

For somebody who once conceded that she would prefer to eat than go to the exercise center, Adele got Pilates and weightlifting in 2019. They are both great aiders in conditioning up and fat loss, which encourages you get the shape you want.

1. Discontinuous fasting – One of the most well-known diet which cycles around a time of fasting and eating. The most widely recognized is 16:8 strategy where you eat for 8 hours and the rest 16 hours is fasting period where you don't eat anything or you can have water if parched. Medical advantages incorporate are decreased aggravation, diminishes muscle to fat ratio stores, battle against malignant growth, lessens cholesterol level, diabetes.

2. Paleo diet – A pattern which centers around nutrition classes, for example, crisp foods grown from the ground, seeds and nuts, lean meat, fish that is wealthy in omega 3, natural oil. Maintain a strategic distance from grains, vegetables, dairy, handled

nourishment, salt, prepared sugar. It would help with weight loss, diminished hunger, controlled sugar levels and circulatory strain.

3. Vegetarian lifestyle – A lifestyle wherein individuals keep away from every one of the items that are gotten from a creature like meat, eggs and all the dairy items however can expend a wide range of organic products, vegetables, grains, vegetables, nuts and seeds. They even limit themselves from gaining any family unit or individual stuff that originates from creatures. The advantages of following such a lifestyle are decreased cardiovascular hazard, diabetes, weight loss and so forth.

4. Without gluten diet – An eating design where you maintain a strategic distance from any nourishment thing that has gluten in it, for example, wheat, rye, grain however separated from this you can appreciate crisp organic product, vegetables, fish, all the dairy item, seeds, nuts, flours which has no gluten present in it. Diminishes muscle to fat ratio stores, swelling, obstruction, improves insusceptible arrangement of the body.

5. Run diet – The Dietary Approaches to Stop Hypertension (DASH) diet is a low sodium, low fat diet. It is wealthy in foods grown from the ground, which guarantees a significant inventory of minerals and nutrients. A scramble diet centers around entire nourishments and rejects all types of handled nourishment.

There are four primary nutrients and minerals found in nourishment that help in advancing rest: tryptophan, magnesium, calcium, and B6. A portion of these substances help the body produce melatonin, the hormone that is liable for directing your circadian mood (rest/wake designs). Magnesium is an incredible mineral that is instrumental in rest and is a characteristic relaxant that deactivates adrenaline. Indeed, it is often alluded to as the rest mineral. Calcium is another mineral that enables the cerebrum to make melatonin. An absence of calcium can make you wake up in the center of the night and experience issues coming back to rest. A few nourishments are normally pressed with these fundamental nutrients and minerals. Here's a rundown:

For tryptophan, have dairy items (milk, low-fat yogurt, cheddar); poultry (turkey, chicken); fish (shrimp, salmon, halibut, fish, sardines, cod); nuts and seeds (flax, sesame, pumpkin, sunflower, cashews, peanuts, almonds, pecans).

For magnesium have dull verdant greens (child spinach, kale, collard greens), wheat germ, fish (salmon, halibut, fish, and mackerel), soybeans, and banana.

For calcium, have low-fat milk, cheeses, yogurt, sardines, fortified grains and soybeans.

For Vitamin B6, have sunflower seeds, pistachio nuts, flaxseed, (fish, salmon, and halibut), and dried prunes. For melatonin, have products of the soil like corn, asparagus, tomatoes, pomegranate, olives, grapes, broccoli, cucumber; grains like rice, grain, moved oats and nuts and seeds.

Nourishments high in fat have been connected to poor, divided rest. Fat triggers the stomach related procedures and causes a development of stomach acids, which while resting can cause distress.

SIRTFOOD DIET THEORY

One more month, another popular diet fanning out quickly over the web.

The most recent eating fever is known as the Sirtfood Diet, and it's grabbing individuals' eye for a couple of reasons. One, it lets you eat stuff like chocolate. Two, it guarantees enormous outcomes immediately—seven pounds in seven days. Also, three, it includes eating "sirtfoods," a mysterious gathering of nourishments that as far as anyone knows contain incredible fat-consuming mixes.

These elements have helped the Sirtfood Diet get on large in England, and it's beginning to advance over the lake. In any case, is the Sirtfood Diet truly a decent method to eat more beneficial? Or on the other hand is it simply one more prevailing fashion of-the-month diet destined to be overlooked?

What are Sirtfoods?

The front of The Sirtfood Diet book calls them "wonder nourishments that turbo-charge weight loss," yet that seems like impervious promoting language. So, what precisely are these marvel nourishments?

Sirtuins (short for Silent Information Regulars, or SIRs) are a class of normally happening proteins in the human body. First found a couple of decades prior, they have energizing capacities, inquire about shows. The exploration contemplates were never performed on genuine individuals (selecting rather for test cylinders or lab creatures), however sirtuins have been found to assume a job in clearing free radicals, lessening irritation, managing our inner clock and forestalling maturing. The exploration has persuaded that sirtuins might be utilized to treat or forestall certain infections, like malignant growth and Type 2 diabetes.

It's additionally been discovered that sirtuins might keep fat cells from copying. The proof isn't firm, yet this is the place the "turbo-charge weight loss" guarantee of the Sirtfood Diet originates from.

Sirtfoods are nourishments rich in sirtuin activators. Sirtuin activators send messages to our DNA to expand the creation of sirtuin proteins. In principle, eating more sirtfoods brings about a more noteworthy creation of sirtuin proteins and every one of the advantages they bring. This is the basic reason of the Sirtfood Diet—eat more sirtfoods, produce more sirtuins and get more fit, decrease aggravation, live more, and so on.

The Diet Plan

The nourishments prescribed by the diet incorporate blueberries, espresso, dull chocolate, arugula, buckwheat, kale, green tea, parsley, additional virgin olive oil, tricks, pecans, onions, turmeric and that's just the beginning.

During the initial three days of the diet, you drink two green squeezes and eat only one dinner for every day. During this time, you are restricted to 1,000 calories for each day. Throughout the following four days, you drink two juices for each day and eat two dinners for every day, while constraining yourself to 1,500 calories for each day. After the principal week and for the following 14 days, you expend an abundance of sirtfoods in three dinners and one juice for every day. Following 21 days, the center changes to "sirtifying" your preferred suppers by embeddings or subbing sirtfoods into plans.

Obviously, the advantages of the Sirtfood Diet come rather rapidly. Numerous dieters report significant weight loss and expanded vitality in simple days.

The Analysis

One clear warning with the Sirtfood Diet is its guarantee of large outcomes in a brief timeframe.

The book has a major red sticker on the spread yelling that members will "lose 7 lbs in 7 days." These kinds of cases regularly demonstrate diets looking to sucker individuals who are edgy to shed pounds, not diets planned for helping individuals make durable lifestyle changes. The "convenient solution" guarantee sets unreasonable desires for dieters, who may be persuaded they can keep on getting in shape at that emotional rate past multi week. Genuine, manageable weight loss is generally accomplished by shedding a couple of pounds seven days.

"I wouldn't be a major aficionado of supporting this kind of eating where it centers around losing a great deal of weight in a short measure of time," says enlisted dietitian Tavis Piattoly, who works as a sustenance advisor to the New Orleans Saints and New Orleans Pelicans. "A great deal of the weight will be water and potentially even muscle tissue."

Additionally, the calorie limitations during the principal week could be out and out risky, particularly if you're a competitor or dynamic individual. Competitors live exceptionally dynamic lifestyles, and young people need significantly a greater number of calories than grown-ups to help legitimate development. Albeit a calorie shortage is the way to getting thinner, too enormous a deficiency can cause issues like constant weariness and absence of core interest. NFL All-Pro guarded end J. J. Watt as of late felt the depleting impacts of a huge calorie shortfall and had to make some genuine diet changes to remain sharp.

Past the principal week, the center shifts from calorie-including to eating dinners high in sirtfoods. This is commonly a nice thought, since the majority of the nourishments associated with the Sirtfood Diet are profoundly nutritious. They're plant-based nourishments, low in calories and high in fiber, protein, nutrients, cancer prevention agents and phytochemicals. They're additionally substantially more difficult to gorge than profoundly handled nourishments.

Nonetheless, the entire "sirtuin activator" thing most likely assumes to a lesser extent a job in the intensity of sirtfoods than the remainder of their nourishing profile. Berries and kale are route preferred for you over treats and chips, whether or not they contain sirtuin activators. If you begin eating more plant-based nourishments, you're going to feel much improved—it's actually that basic.

The Verdict

We praise the Sirtfood Diet for its emphasis on eating more plant-based nourishments, however it's unquestionably not an ideal diet.

The underlying calorie limitations are unreasonably exacting for some individuals, and the guarantee of seven pounds of weight loss in the initial seven days is anything but a solid methodology. The huge spotlight on sirtuins is likewise somewhat odd, since the exploration on sirtuins (and specifically, their job in weight the executives) is as yet starter. The sirtfoods remembered for the Sirtfood Diet are for the most part sound plant-based nourishments high in an assortment of supplements. We're speculating a great many different supplements and mixes in these nourishments (the majority of which are more well-examined than sirtuin activators) are the genuine motivation behind why individuals are revealing sirtfoods assist them with feeling and look better. A lot of sound nourishments are excluded from the Sirtfood Diet and maintaining a strategic distance from them exclusively considering that is absolutely superfluous.

If you're hoping to get more fit, your initial step ought to be to eliminate refined sugar items (pop, treats, and so on.) and excursions to the drive-through. Supplant those nourishments with plant-based alternatives and drink more water. If you're eating the correct sorts of nourishments, the amount you're eating shouldn't be a significant issue.

You should likewise meet with a wellbeing proficient or enlisted dietitian. They can customize an arrangement for you as opposed to utilizing the "one-size-fits-all" approach numerous trend diets depend on. What's more, recollect—gradual advancement is often the most secure and the most manageable approach to get more fit.

The Sirtfood Diet: the most recent in a not insignificant rundown of BS faddy diets customers, companions, and family, have sent me for my expert scrutinize. I figured that if they were asking, then others must have questions as well. This is a quite extensive book so here's the TL:DR - this diet is false, don't get the book, work with a qualified nutritionist.

Still with me? How about we separate it.

Most importantly, we have to comprehend what sirtfoods are, and to get that, we have to realize what sirtuins are. You all prepared for a little science? Here we go.

Sirtuins are a gathering of proteins known as Silent Information Regulators, or SIRs. They were found in people a couple of decades prior, and have been forcefully examined from that point forward, for the most part at a subcellular level or in lab creatures (for example very few examinations in genuine human individuals). This has driven researchers to make energizing disclosures about the job of these proteins in securing metabolic wellbeing, including: guideline of our natural tickers (otherwise known as circadian cadence), lessening irritation, wiping up free radicals that can make harm DNA, assisting with ensuring the honesty of our DNA and keep it from untimely maturing; therefore SIRs may assume a significant job in counteraction of Alzheimer's. Researchers likewise figure they might be significant in securing against (and perhaps treating) illness like sort 2 diabetes, cardiovascular sicknesses like respiratory failures and stroke, and even a few tumors. Really energizing stuff, isn't that so? Right! Be that as it may, it's imperative to state that, in spite of the fact that these discoveries are promising, they're 1) reductionist in nature (for example we don't simply eat just sirtfoods) and 2) we don't have numerous examinations in people yet.

Anyway, sirtuins have been embroiled in keeping fat cells from copying, a wonder known as adipogenesis (fat cells being the latin for fat) (lol jk, yet fat means fat). It was now that the creators of 'The Sirtfood Diet' heard a 'KA-CHING' and saw little $$ drifting before them.

Along these lines, the hypothesis is then, that specific nourishments can upregulate the declaration of the SIR qualities. Every one of that implies is that sure nourishments send messages to our DNA to instruct them to make a greater amount of the sirtuin proteins. In this way, more sirtfoods=more sir proteins. Alright? It's somewhat more muddled than that, yet you get the thought.

The creators of TSD, made this a stride further and essentially arrived at the resolution that if you make a diet up of a lot of these alleged 'sirtfoods' you'll not just impact individuals' fat cells and make them free a lot of weight, yet they'll adequately get undying all the while.

The diet is separated into three phases as clarified here, yet to sum things up: The "Hyper Success Phase" (motivated naming there folks), whereby dieters are limited to 1000kcals every day made up of three sirtfood green juices and a sirtfood rich dinner. For three days in a row. Stage two then, gets an extra 500kcal, on the grounds that you dump one of the juices and supplant it with real nourishment - sirtfoods, however. Recollect that, it's significant. Toward the week's end you go into the support period of 3 sirtfood rich dinners in addition to a sirtfood juice.

The creators put this diet under a magnifying glass in their first class, private individuals rec center, where members (n=40) got instructional courses with a fitness coach and were under the creators' master healthful direction. They paid around £1,500 for the benefit as well. I think we'd all concur this was a thorough and replicable examination, no?

To be completely forthright: I have not perused the book (hello, nobody sent me a development duplicate and nobody's paying me for composing this poo). Anyway, in view of what I can gather from the popularpress (and yes I realize it would not stand up as an authentic source in the court of science, yet simply stay with me), here are every one of the issues I have with The Sirtfood Diet. An answer, if you will.

7lbs in 7 days

In this way, the large case from TSD is that you can lose 7lbs in 7 days. Goggins and Matten guarantee that their diet isn't about weight loss, it's about wellbeing, however this 7 out of 7 is key to their showcasing technique. It's spread all around the title page of the book FFS. In addition to the fact that this is somewhat weight loss impractical, sensational, and unfortunate, it tends to be mentally harming to set somebody up with this sort of ridiculous desire for the diet. 1-2lbs every week is the suggestion for weight loss. It doesn't occur without any forethought, it's moderate and steady and hella baffling. My speculation is that it didn't all go on medium-term, so we have to have practical assumptions regarding losing it as well.

Calorie Restriction Vs Sirtfoods

The second thing that truly bothers me about this diet is that it's difficult to uncouple the impacts of sirtfoods from calorie limitation. That is to say, folks, where was the benchmark group in your 'study'? Please, that resembles, fundamental crap. When you radically limit calories to half of what an individual ought to typically devour, odds are, you will get thinner. I couldn't care less if it's 1000ckals of bananas or scones, you gon' get thinner, child. Exactly at the expectation of trolls; yes, I know weight loss is more mind boggling than that. Calories in =calories out is a gross oversimplification. I additionally realize that long haul calorie limitation can bring about metabolic stagnation, which is the reason, I generally suggest you work with a qualified proficient when attempting to shift a few lbs. However, you know, when all is said in done.

Are sirtfoods truly even all that?

Above all else, I truly despise the term sirtfoods, it's an absolute misnomer. The nourishments prescribed by the sirtfood diets: kale, green tea, blueberries, espresso, dull chocolate, red wine, rocket/arugula, parsley don't really contain sirtuins. Certain phytonutrients (plant supplements) in the nourishments advance or animate the generation of these proteins (recall out little science talk?). Try not to misunderstand me, generally these nourishments are SUPER solid (the red wine is faulty, I mean, liquor is actually a poison). Be that as it may, stop and think for a minute, sirtfoods contain a shitload of wellbeing advancing phytonutrients. I'm talking ≥10,000 different mixes - not simply the ones that advance sirtuin action (polyphenols). We have bioflavonoids, carotenoids, retinols, isoflavones, genistein, lycopene, sulphoraphones, and, you get the image. Be that as it may, these mixes aren't select to sirtfoods, nor do sirtfoods hold the rights to SIR advancing action. The fact of the matter is, eat a wide assortment of plant based nourishments, similar to natural product, veg, and beans to get all the great phytochemicals, max your digestion, and forestall malady. As it were, sirtfoods aren't all that, and thank to Goggins and his bud, they will be super spenny in the shops now as well.

Sirtify your life

The creators have offered expressions about how all you gotta do is add a sirtfood bend to your preferred dishes. Right... Things being what they are, imagine a scenario where your preferred dinner is singed chicken. Or on the other hand steak and chips? What these two dipshits need to get across is that nourishments high in fat and protein produce glycotoxins (or propelled glycation final results if you need to get extravagant). Glycotoxins suppress sirtuin movement. Some are created naturally by the body, yet for the most part they originate from the diet. The greatest dietary sources are chicken, hamburger, pork and fish, especially if flame broiled or singed. What's more, a few researchers propose that these are (in any event in part) answerable for the 3X more serious danger of dementia among meat eaters than among veggie lovers. They've likewise been involved in type 2 diabetes chance. So why then, are these folks instructing you to eat chicken curry, and bean stew con carne? A side of kale isn't going to fix that, you need to take a gander at the nourishments you eat all in all.

Sirtfoods are by all account not the only method to expand your sirtuin action

Sirtuins are likewise created through caloric limitation and exercise.

Concentrate on sirtjuices?

I've just spoken finally concerning why juice scrubs are moronic, so I'll keep this brief. I think there is space in the diet for individuals to incorporate green squeeze that is vegetable based. I don't think 2-3 juices, as swaps for genuine wholefood dinners is sound or mindful sustenance guidance.

In the interminable expressions of Michael Pollan: "Eat nourishment. For the most part plants. Not all that much", and if you need assistance exploring that message, get yourself a nutritionist who can jump aboard with it.

SIRTFOOD SCIENCE. ITS IMPLICATION WITH MUSCLE MASS, DISEASE, FAT AND DIET

Since days of yore, people have been intrigued by the quest for the legendary wellspring of youth. Quick forward to the twenty-first century and sirtfood science nothing has changed, with gigantic scientific intrigue presently centered around a group of digestion managing qualities called sirtuin, and their strong activities which can on a very basic level change how our phones work. These intense qualities assist us with consuming fat, become fitter and fight off infection, and eventually could be the nearest we ever find a good pace the clock.

Be that as it may, regardless of whether we like to consider them 'thin qualities' or 'Diminish Pan qualities' as the media likes to coin them, what makes sirtuins extraordinary is their capacity to switch our cells into an endurance mode. They do this by enacting an incredible reusing process called autophagy, which gets out cell burn through and garbage that develops after some time and is known to cause 'inflammaging'. The impacts of this restoration procedure are great: our cells come back to a progressively energetic state where aggravation is extinguished, fat consuming increments and we by and by feel like we did in our prime.

Which asks the million dollar question: how might we actuate sirtuins and receive their striking rewards? There are two entrenched techniques: fasting and exercise. However, as anybody will let you know, both can be overwhelming, and often not good with our occupied and requesting twenty-first century lifestyle. Their ruins are additionally notable. The same number of will authenticate, reducing calories makes us tired and 'hangry' (that impressively upsetting blend of eager and furious), and in the more extended term can disintegrate muscle and cause digestion to stagnate. With respect to work out, the sum should have been powerful for weight loss is skirting on the enormous.

In any case, imagine a scenario in which there was a third, less exhausting, way, a way that nature had constantly proposed for us.

In 2013 the consequences of one of the greatest distinct advantages by the way we comprehend nourishment was distributed. It was called PREDIMED, the biggest, best-directed sustenance study did in the cutting edge time. Done on right around 7,500 individuals, PREDIMED posed a straightforward inquiry: how did a Mediterranean-style diet enhanced with liberal additional virgin olive oil or nuts (particularly pecans) contrast with a progressively ordinary present day diet? The outcomes were exceptional. Following 5 years, coronary illness and diabetes were cut by a surprising 30%, joined by significant decreases in irritation just as the danger of heftiness. Yet, what was generally striking about this examination was still to come. Upon further examination, it happened that there was no significant difference between the two gatherings in the quantity of calories, fat or sugars they expended. These are all the standard estimates we use when we decide how sound a diet is. There was something by and large different continuing, something that presently couldn't seem to be considered by cutting edge nourishment.

Plant nourishments – like additional virgin olive oil and pecans – contain normal mixes called polyphenols, which examine now shows have monstrous medical advantages. When analysts breaking down PREDIMED explored polyphenol utilization the outcomes were faltering. Over simply the multiyear time span the individuals who devoured the most elevated levels of polyphenols had 37% less passings contrasted with the individuals who expended the least.

Be that as it may, not all polyphenols are equivalent. For example, an investigation of very nearly 3,000 twins found that a higher admission of just certain polyphenols was connected with less muscle versus fat and a more advantageous dissemination of fat in the body. Specific polyphenols are without a doubt a shelter for remaining thin and sound, yet which polyphenols are the best? Might it be able to be those that examination has indicated have the capacity to turn on our sirtuin qualities? Exactly the same ones actuated by fasting and exercise?

The pharmaceutical business has rushed to hop on this thought, contributing tremendous measures of cash to change over sirtuin initiating supplements into panacea drugs. Glaxo Smith Kline made a major mix when they paid just about a billion dollars for the rights to inquire about the nourishment supplement resveratrol and form it into a sirtuin initiating drug. Be that as it may, they succumbed to the entanglement of detaching a solitary supplement and giving it at pharmaceutical portions, when research shows that the advantages originate from a collaboration of supplements expended at dosages that it is conceivable to accomplish through dietary sources.

Many will have known about the most well-known diabetes medicate metformin, and many perusing this will either take it or know somebody who does. What you can be sure of is that it has common plant sources, originating from the French lilac plant and was utilized as far, thinking back to the 1800s to treat diabetes. Furthermore, while most well-known medications are related with considerable reactions restricting their utilization, metformin has the award of being the principal FDA endorsed medication to be examined for expanding life, so strong are its medical advantages. What's more, what causes such massive advantage? We currently realize it is on the grounds that metformin doesn't follow up on glucose or macronutrients straightforwardly however works by actuating the sirtuin quality pathway.

Incomprehensibly, while the pharmaceutical business has been everywhere throughout the sensational capacity of plants to work at a hereditary level to change wellbeing, it's a thought that has been on the whole overlooked in the nourishment world.

Specialists of the Sirtfood Diet set out to find which nourishments contained the most significant level of the specific polyphenols that had been appeared in pharmaceutical screening concentrates to actuate sirtuin qualities. This finished in the identification of the best 20 Sirtfoods, which we painstakingly set up into an exceptional diet. This included additional virgin olive oil and pecans, much the same as in PREDIMED; just as arugula, red onions, strawberries, red wine, cocoa, chillies, turmeric, green tea and espresso among other. When street tried this diet delivered staggering outcomes. Members lost, by and large, 7lbs in 7 days, while either keeping up or in any event, expanding their bulk. Best surprisingly detailed inclination extraordinary; overflowing with vitality, dozing better and with prominent upgrades in their skin.

While this spoke to an incredible launch, it was the long haul results that really indicated the intensity of these plant nourishments as individuals lost in the scope of 20 to 50 pounds more than 12 weeks. This included numerous free tests, including as of late a distrustful specialist testing it on national TV, with his patient losing a stunning 22 pounds in an unimportant a month. However, to concentrate just on weight loss is an insult to our clinicians and the stunning nourishments that work at the most profound hereditary degree of our cells to stop irritation and maturing. The Sirtfood Diet clinicians acknowledged they had found something really unique with the life-changing wellbeing changes, including individuals who turned around diabetes, coronary illness and auto-invulnerable ailments and had the option to surrender their prescriptions. Until this point in time, countless individuals around the globe have now encountered the incredible impacts of the Sirtfood Diet and the tributes keep on flooding in.

Undoubtedly the advantages of a diet based around these nourishments gives us that wellbeing isn't characterized by calorie forgetting about, removing carbs, or banishing fat. Nature never expected us to be solid dependent on what we cut out. Or maybe, nature planned for us to receive the rewards of a long and solid life by enjoying its unmatched nourishment drug store.

Not many things are so profoundly tainted by prevailing fashions, fakes and pretense as sustenance. Accordingly, it is through a viewpoint of sound distrust that we should see any new diet. The most recent to stand out as truly newsworthy is the Sirtfood diet which, if we are to fully trust claims, will help with weight loss just as offering different advantages, for example, "animating restoration and cell fix".

For the unenlightened, this most recent diet is based around utilization of nourishments which may associate with a group of proteins known as sirtuin proteins, or SIRT1 - SIRT7. Adding to the diet's undoubted request is the way that the best sources as far as anyone knows incorporate red wine and chocolate, just as citrus natural products, blueberries and kale. During the initial three days, calorie admission is constrained (1,000 calories for every day) and comprises of three Sirtfood green juices, in addition to an ordinary dinner rich in "Sirtfoods". On days four to seven, calorie admission is expanded (1,500 calories) and comprises of two juices and two dinners. Past that the suggestion is to eat a fair diet rich in sirtuin nourishments, alongside further green juices. Prawns and salmon likewise include in the dinner plans.

It sounds scrumptious – and sirtuins are surely ensnared in a wide scope of cell forms including digestion, maturing and circadian mood. The diet is additionally situated to a limited extent, on calorie limitation. The nutritionists behind this propose the diet "impacts the body's capacity to consume fat and lifts the metabolic framework".

The Diet Decoded

So, what do we think about this diet? From a scientific point of view, the appropriate response is practically nothing. Sirtuins add to guideline of fat and glucose digestion considering changes in vitality levels. They may likewise have an impact in the impact of calorie limitation on upgrades in maturing. This is maybe by means of sirtuins' consequences for vigorous (or mitochondrial) digestion, bringing down of responsive oxygen species (free radicals) and increments in cancer prevention agent catalysts.

Moreover, inquire about recommends that transgenic mice with more elevated levels of SIRT6 live significantly longer than wild-type mice, and that changes in SIRT6 articulation might be applicable in maturing of some human skin cells. SIRT2 likewise has been shown to moderate metazoan (yeast) maturing.

It sounds great and the diet makes them gleam surveys, however none of this speaks to convincing scientific proof of the Sirtfood Diet effects affecting genuine individuals. It would be a colossal over-extrapolation to expect that lab investigate directed on mice, yeast and human immature microorganisms has any bearing on true wellbeing results – corrupted as they are by a huge number of puzzling factors.

The Science of Weight Loss

Surely the diet will seem to work for certain individuals. In any case, scientific confirmation of any diet's triumphs is an altogether different issue. Obviously, the perfect investigation to think about the viability of a diet on weight loss (or some other result, for example, maturing) would require an adequately enormous example – delegate of the populace we are keen on – and irregular distribution to a treatment or control gathering. Results would then be checked over an enough timeframe with severe command over puzzling factors, for example, different practices that may decidedly or adversely influence the results of enthusiasm (smoking, for example, or work out).

This examination would be constrained by techniques, for example, self-revealing and memory, however, would go some approach to finding the viability of this diet. Research of this nature, be that as it may, doesn't exist and we ought to therefore be wary when deciphering essential science – all things considered, human cells in a tissue culture dish presumably respond differently to the phones in a living individual.

Further uncertainty is thrown over this diet when we think about a portion of the specific cases. Losses of seven pounds in a single week are ridiculous and are probably not going to reflect changes to muscle to fat ratio. For the initial three days, dieters expend around 1000 kcal every day – around 40–half of what a great many people require. This will bring about a fast loss of glycogen (a put away type of starch) from skeletal muscle and the liver.

Yet, for each gram of put away glycogen we additionally store roughly 2.7 grams of water, and water is overwhelming. So, for all the lost glycogen, we likewise lose going with water – and henceforth weight. Furthermore, diets that are too prohibitive are difficult to follow and bring about increments in hunger invigorating hormones, for example, ghrelin. Weight (glycogen and water) will therefore come back to typical if the desire to eat wins out.

As a rule, use of the scientific technique to the investigation of sustenance is difficult. It is often unrealistic to do fake treatment controlled preliminaries with any level of natural legitimacy, and the wellbeing results that we are often keen on happen over numerous years, making research configuration testing. Besides, considers in huge populaces rely upon shockingly shortsighted and guileless information assortment strategies, for example, memory and self-announcing, which produce famously inconsistent information. Against this foundation commotion, nourishment look into has a difficult activity.

Is There A Quick Fix?

Sadly, not. Sensationalized features and often hyperbolic portrayal of scientific information brings about the apparently unlimited debates about what – and how much – we ought to eat, further fuelling our fixation on a "convenient solution" or marvel fix, which in itself is an endemic social issue.

For the reasons sketched out, the Sirtfood diet ought to be entrusted to the prevailing fashion heap – at any rate from a scientific point of view. In light of the proof we have, to recommend in any case is, best case scenario fake and even under the least favorable conditions deceiving and harming to the authentic points of general wellbeing procedure. The diet is probably not going to offer any profit to populaces confronting a scourge of diabetes, sneaking in the shadow of corpulence. As expressed plainly by others, uncommon diets don't work and dieting all in all is certainly not a general wellbeing answer for social orders where the greater part of grown-ups are overweight.

By and by, the best technique is long haul conduct change joined with political and natural impact, focused on expanded physical movement and some type of cognizant command over what we eat. It is anything but a convenient solution, yet it will work.

A diet that underlines dull chocolate, red wine, kale, berries, and espresso? It either seems like the most ideal street to wellbeing and weight loss, or unrealistic. However, pause, it shows signs of improvement: According to the makers of the Sirtfood Diet, these and other supposed "sirtfoods" are indicated to enact the components constrained by your body's characteristic "thin qualities" to assist you with consuming fat and get more fit.

Bragging a rundown flavorful nourishment, you presumably as of now love, and supported by reports that Adele utilized it to get in shape in the wake of having a child, the Sirtfood Diet sounds naturally engaging.

Be that as it may, not to destroy your chocolate-and-red-wine high here, yet the science doesn't really bolster the diet's greatest cases. Which isn't to say that eating sirtfoods is an ill-conceived notion . . . yet, similarly as with all diets that sound unrealistic, you should take a gander at this one with genuine examination. This is what you have to think about what sirtfoods can and can't accomplish for you.

As a matter of first importance, what the hell is a sirtfood?

Created by U.K. sustenance experts Aidan Goggins and Glen Matten, the Sirtfood Diet underlines plant-based nourishments that are known "sirtuin activators." Basically, when you nosh on the arrangement's key fixings, you animate the proteins encoded for by the SIRT1 quality, which Goggins and Matten have named "the thin quality."

SIRT1 and sirtuin proteins are accepted to assume a job in maturing and life span, which might be identified with the defensive impacts of calorie limitation. The case behind the Sirtfood Diet is that sure nourishments can actuate these sirt-intervened pathways sans the limitation, and consequently "switch on your muscle to fat ratio's consuming forces, supercharge weight loss, and assist fight with offing infection."

Alongside red wine, dull chocolate, berries, espresso, and kale, sirtuin-advancing nourishments incorporate matcha green tea, additional virgin olive oil, pecans, parsley, red onions, soy, and turmeric (a.k.a. phenomenal flavors and go-to solid treats).

There's some science behind the cases of sirtfoods' advantages, yet it's exceptionally constrained and rather disputable.

The science on the sirt boondocks is still very new. There are contemplates investigating the SIRT1 quality's job in maturing and life span, in maturing related weight addition and maturing related illness, and in shielding the heart from aggravation brought about by a high-fat diet. In any case, the examination is restricted to work done in test tubes and on mice, which isn't adequate proof to state that sirtuin-boosting nourishments can have weight loss or against maturing capacities in an absolutely real human body.

Brooke Alpert, R.D., creator of The Sugar Detox, says there's exploration to recommend that the weight-control advantages of sirtfoods may come to some degree from the polyphenol-cancer prevention agent resveratrol, often advertised as a component in red wine. "All things considered, it is difficult to devour enough red wine to get benefits," she says, noticing that she does much of the time recommend resveratrol enhancements to her customers.

Also, some nourishment specialists aren't psyched about the manner in which the Sirtfood Diet plan works.

According to top dietitians who've evaluated the arrangement, the Sirtfood Diet is feeling the loss of some significant components for a sound, adjusted routine. Goggins and Matten's diet plan includes three stages: a couple of days at 1,000 calories for each day, made up of one sirtfood-overwhelming dinner and green squeezes; a couple of long periods of two sirtfood suppers and two squeezes per day, for an aggregate of 1,500 calories; and a fourteen day support period of sirt-y suppers and juices.

Keri Gans, R.D., creator of The Small Change Diet, says that she's "not wild about anything that runs in stages." Usually, the shorter stages make a hardship organize, which just prompts gorging later on. "When you're limiting, anybody will get in shape toward the beginning of a diet," she clarifies. "However, we can't continue that eating design long haul."

According to Lauren Blake, R.D., a dietitian at the Ohio State University Wexner Medical Center, when you're hydrating and squeezing a great deal without a huge amount of calorie consumption, weight loss is normal, "however it's ordinarily liquid loss," she clarifies. So, while one may shed beats on the diet, it's probably going to be impermanent and might have nothing to do with sirtuins by any means.

The decision? Sirtfoods are incredible to have in your diet, however they shouldn't be all you have.

There's positively no explanation you can't include some sirtfoods into your eating plan, says Alpert. "I think there are some truly fascinating things here, similar to the red wine, dull chocolate, matcha—I love these things," she says. "I love mentioning to individuals what to concentrate on rather than what to nix from their diet." If it tastes liberal and it's solid in little amounts, why not?

Gans says she's an enthusiast of a ton of the nourishments on the sirt list, including staples of the Mediterranean Diet—the highest quality level of scientifically-supported smart dieting—like olive oil, berries, and red wine. "I can get behind nourishments rich in polyphenols and cancer prevention agents," she says.

Blake concurs that there's bounty to adore about the nourishments remembered for the diet, particularly the stylish fixings like turmeric and matcha that vibe crisp and help make eating fun and intriguing. "I'm seeing a great deal of plant-based nourishments that truly sparkle, and are loaded up with phytonutrients," she says. "Those are calming, and bravo."

Be that as it may, all the nourishment specialists recommend balancing the diet with some lean protein and sound fats, for example, progressively nuts and seeds, avocado, and greasy fish like salmon. Stir up your plate of mixed greens game, as well, with more kinds of veggies, spinach, and romaine lettuce notwithstanding the kale and red onions. Main concern? A large portion of the sirtfoods are An OK to eat and solid for you, yet simply don't depend on the diet to enact any "thin quality" right now.

With Muscles

For what reason is SIRT1 viewed as a 'life span' quality? SirT1 is the mammalian ortholog of yeast Sir2, a chemical that is engaged with protein deacetylation, which was first described as a significant controller of life length right now, hence in higher eukaryotes (Longo and Kennedy, 2006). Be that as it may, regardless of whether SirT1 is related with an augmentation of the life length of human cells involves some discussion (Michishita et al., 2005). SirT1 substrates and transcriptional/epigenetic co-factors make up a great and continually developing rundown, including, among others, PGC-1α, HNF4α, p53, FOXOs, PPARγ, NF-κB, Ku70, PCAF, MyoD, MEF2, STAT3, HSF1, Smad7, Suv39h1, Ezh2, nucleomethylin, eNoSC and different histones (Nemoto et al., 2004; Nemoto et al., 2005; Rodgers et al., 2005; Kume et al., 2007; Grummt and Ladurner, 2008; Finkel et al., 2009; Nie et al., 2009; Vaquero and Reinberg, 2009; Westerheide et al., 2009). SirT1 impacts various procedures that are significant to cell reasonability, for example, quality quieting or enactment, apoptosis, stress opposition, senescence, vitality equalization, and lipid and glucose digestion. Later rich work on SirT1 knockout mouse early stage fibroblasts (MEFs) and undeveloped undifferentiated cells demonstrated that SirT1 movement impacts practically on the circadian clock (Asher et al., 2008; Nakahata et al., 2008) and on genome (chromatin) strength (Oberdoerffer et al., 2008; Wang et al., 2008), and an incorporated picture of SirT1-subordinate enemy of malignant growth and hostile to maturing impacts is simply rising (Jung-Hynes and Ahmad, 2009; Liu et al., 2009).

A few systems that are fit for initiating sirtuin enzymatic action have been appeared to build life length. Old style activators of SirT1 incorporate the polyphenol resveratrol (contained in red grapes and green tea) (Howitz et al., 2003), just as a routine of caloric limitation (CR) (Cohen et al., 2004). CR, characterized in mice as a decrease in nourishment admission of 30%–half contrasted and creatures encouraged not obligatory, is a very notable intercession that upgrades life span in research facility creatures. CR may really build life length by setting off an unpredictable exchange of flagging particles, including SirT1, yet in addition AMP-enacted protein kinase (AMPK), forkhead box O translation factors (FOXOs), mammalian objective of rapamycin (mTOR), and the proportion of NAD+ to NADH (Cantó and Auwerx, 2009b). Thus, resveratrol impacts on extra cell pathways, likely inferable from its substance nature as a protein-restricting polyphenol. Inferable from the pleiotropic beneficial outcomes of SirT1 on the strength of life forms, the pharmaceutical business has demonstrated a developing enthusiasm for creating exacerbates that can balance SirT1 action (Lavu et al., 2008).

Right now, will limit our emphasis on the job of SirT1 movement in two striated muscle tissues of early stage mesodermic root, skeletal and heart muscle, which oversee major procedures, for example, glucose and lipid digestion, physical action, and drive of blood around the circulatory framework, with a specific consideration regarding important SirT1-specific mouse models. Perusers who are keen on different sirtuins (SirT2–SirT7) or in other tissue-specific SirT1 mice models are alluded to the ongoing phenomenal audits by Finkel et al. what's more, (Guarente, 2007; Finkel et al., 2009).

Given the advancements accessible to control the mouse genome (van der Weyden et al., 2003), and the high level of homology among murine and human genomes, the mouse is viewed as the head living being for demonstrating human pathologies. Utilizing the mouse as a model life form gives the plausibility of producing loss-of-capacity and addition of-work freaks of sickness up-and-comer proteins, even in a contingent (tissue-specific) or potentially inducible way. Right now, learned in 2003 that, when produced in an ingrained hereditary foundation, entire body SirT1 knockout (KO) mice conveying two invalid alleles of Sirt1 kick the bucket prenatally or during the early postnatal period, with neurological and heart contortions (Cheng et al., 2003; McBurney et al., 2003). This focuses to a vital job for dynamic SirT1 in homeostasis. Be that as it may, in outbred foundations, entire body SirT1 KO produces reasonable mice with differing phenotypes, for example, flawed gametogenesis and sterility (McBurney et al., 2003; Coussens et al., 2008); an immune system like condition (Sequeira et al., 2008); and a hindrance in acquiring profits by the positive CR-initiated metabolic impacts (Boily et al., 2008). These discoveries feature the significance of considering the effect of hereditary foundation inconstancy when breaking down murine phenotypes. On the other hand, entire body bacterial artificial chromosome (BAC)- driven transgenic (Tg) overexpression of SirT1 in mice, even at moderate levels (~ twofold to triple), has been unequivocally demonstrated to be valuable, prompting an expansion in vitality productivity and forestalling metabolic harm (Banks et al., 2008; Pfluger et al.,

2008). SirT1 overexpression is therefore thought to look like intently the valuable phenotype prompted by CR (Bordone et al., 2007). Given that CR is an exceptionally effective methodology to invert both the clinical highlights of metabolic disorders, for example, heftiness and insulin opposition in people (Opie, 2009), and the CR-like phenotypes of SirT1-overexpressing mice, this proof recommends that new SirT1-enacting mixes could be helpful for the future administration of patients experiencing metabolic unsettling influences.

The enzymatic response did by SirT1, its objectives, including transcriptional co-variables, and ward natural procedures. SirT1 protein substrate(s) is spoken to as a string of blue square shapes, with acetylated (Ac) lysine (K) deposits. Utilizing NAD+ as a co-factor, SirT1 can deacetylate histones, and atomic and cytoplasmic proteins on specific K deposits. This response produces a deacetylated protein, nicotinamide and O-acetyl-ADP-ribose (OAADPR). SirT1 action can be upgraded by caloric limitation (CR) and by the polyphenol resveratrol, influencing numerous formatives, physiological and obsessive procedures, and at last supporting wellbeing and expanding life span.

What occurs if SirT1 is artificially controlled in mouse skeletal or heart muscle cells? Skeletal muscle specific SirT1 Tg or KO mice models have not yet been accounted for, however the impacts of SirT1 have been considered broadly in skeletal muscle cells. A unique report utilizing refined murine myotubes and human essential skeletal muscle cells exhibited that SirT1 overexpression curbs the muscle transcriptional controller MyoD (Fulco et al., 2003). As an outcome, the creation of a few transcripts including those encoding myogenin and muscle contractile proteins was blocked, and muscle differentiation, which was checked as a diminished combination of myoblasts into myotubes, was seriously repressed (Fulco et al., 2003). The proportion of NAD+ to NADH and the redox state are personally connected to supplement accessibility in muscle cells, and a rich follow-up of this workplaces SirT1 at the junction between the two. If refined myoblasts are presented to glucose limitation, SirT1 action is upgraded through AMPK-subordinate guideline of NAM phosphoribosyl transferase (NAMPT), the rate-constraining compound that is answerable for NAD+ turnover, and this squares differentiation into myotubes (Fulco et al., 2008). Also, in refined myotubes, the nearness of SirT1 was demonstrated to be fundamental for the phone self-sufficient change from glucose use to unsaturated fat oxidation within the sight of a low glucose fixation; this adaptable metabolic reaction happens during CR and is commonly debilitated during metabolic sicknesses (Gerhart-Hines et al., 2007). These and other fundamental in vitro examinations in this way revealed a key job for SirT1 in molding muscle cell digestion and differentiation by utilitarian association with different controllers of cell vitality stores, for example, AMPK and peroxisome proliferator-actuated receptor gamma (PPARγ) coactivator-1 alpha (PGC-1α) (Nemoto et al., 2005; Lagouge et al., 2006; Gerhart-Hines et al., 2007; Amat et al., 2009; Cantó and Auwerx, 2009a). The field presently anticipates skeletal muscle specific SirT1 Tg or KO mice models, which would affirm, in vivo, the job of SirT1 in the differentiation, digestion and contractile capacity of this tissue at the degree of an entire living being.

Conversely, two heart limited Tg SirT1 mouse models, acquired by utilizing the tissue specific α-myosin substantial chain (α-MHC) advertiser, have been depicted (Alcendor et al., 2007; Pillai et al., 2008). In one examination, low to direct (about triple to eightfold) SirT1 overexpression proficiently shielded mice from paraquat-initiated cardiovascular pressure and apoptosis and postponed the beginning of age-subordinate heart dysfunctions (Alcendor et al., 2007). Then again, more prominent increments in SirT1 levels (around 13-overlap) prompted oxidative pressure and apoptosis, at last prompting cardiomyopathy and diminished endurance (Alcendor et al., 2007). This was the principal report to present the 'hormesis' idea, implying that SirT1 initiation – relying upon its degree – can be either valuable or pernicious in the heart. A subsequent report demonstrated that Tg heart-limited SirT1 overexpression upregulated α-MHC levels and ensured against the switch in cardiovascular MHC isoform articulation (α to β) that is initiated by 6-propyl-2-thiouracil (PTU), an intense antithyroid medication (Pillai et al., 2008).

In equal, in vitro discoveries from refined or essential cardiomyocyte models extended our comprehension of the cardioprotective impacts of the life span protein SirT1 and expanded NAD+ accessibility, including the expanded protection from ischemia/reperfusion-prompted oxidative pressure (Hsu et al., 2009; Rane et al., 2009), angiotensin II-subordinate hypertrophy (Pillai et al., 2006) and apoptosis (Alcendor et al., 2004; Pillai et al., 2005), in this manner strengthening the view that pharmacological SirT1 enactment may be advantageous for the treatment of heart illnesses (Hsu et al., 2008; Lavu et al., 2008; Borradaile et al., 2009).

Restorative territories that will likely profit by SirT1 look into are (1) the control of diminished bulk and (2) muscle recovery upon damage. To begin with, bulk is decreased during a state of decay, (for example, because of starvation, immobilization or treatment with glucocorticoids) or cachexia, which prompts muscle squandering inferable from expanded protein catabolism (McKinnell and Rudnicki, 2004; Mourkioti and Rosenthal, 2005). Muscle-specific RING finger protein 1 (MuRF1) and MAFbx/atrogin-1, which are E3 ubiquitin ligases engaged with proteasome-interceded proteolysis of muscle proteins, are transcriptionally constrained by NF-κB and FOXOs, individually (Glass, 2005). Since SirT1 adjusts both NF-κB and FOXOs, working together with controlling MyoD and myocyte enhancer factor-2 (MEF2), it might likewise control bulk during damage. Moreover, SirT1 controls angiogenesis and vasculogenesis during improvement (Potente et al., 2007; Potente and Dimmeler, 2008); in any case, its regenerative potential in different tissues is obscure. This is a functioning field of examination in skeletal and heart muscle illnesses since these tissues were for quite some time considered 'post-mitotic' and therefore have a restricted regenerative limit after maturing, harm, skeletal muscle dystrophy or cardiovascular infarct.

As of late, numerous endeavors have depended on the portrayal of skeletal or heart muscle-specific stem and additionally satellite cells that, once enrolled, may add to fixing harmed tissues. Since it has been suggested that SirT1 may likewise impact the ancestry/cell-destiny choices of foundational microorganisms by detecting redox status (Machida and Booth, 2004; Mantel and Broxmeyer, 2008), it is possible that SirT1 may likewise impact the regenerative capability of skeletal muscle and the heart, by influencing the initiation, proliferation and differentiation of their separate grown-up immature microorganisms. Two lines of proof help this speculation. To start with, class I and II histone deacetylase inhibitors end up being advantageous for strong practical recuperation in dystrophic mouse models (Minetti et al., 2006; Colussi et al., 2008). In any case, we disregard whether adjustment of SirT1 action in dystrophic skeletal muscle may enhance the illness. Pharmacological actuation/hindrance of SirtT1 together with consolidated hereditary investigations utilizing restrictive satellite cell-specific SirT1 Tg/KO and dystrophic, (for example, MDX) mice models would without a doubt shed light on this issue. Second, locally acting isoforms of insulin development factor-1 (IGF-1) have incredible fix and regenerative impacts in harmed skeletal and heart muscle tissue (Musaro et al., 1999; Musaro et al., 2001; Barton et al., 2002; Winn et al., 2002; Musarò et al., 2004; Mourkioti and Rosenthal, 2005; Schulze et al., 2005; Pelosi et al., 2007). Strikingly, IGF-1 and SirT1 share downstream flagging targets, for example, FOXOs, in skeletal myocytes and cardiomyocytes. It has been accounted for that flowing IGF-1 neutralized SirT1 action (Cohen et al., 2004). Additionally, the degrees of coursing IGF-1 are brought down upon caloric limitation (Huffman et al., 2008). Consequently, SirT1 and flowing IGF-1 assume inverse natural jobs in life span (Longo, 2009), however it is obscure how muscle and heart SirT1 action impacts on the regenerative capability of discrete IGF-1 isoforms, acting locally or fundamentally. We propose that significant advances right now will be accomplished by the consolidated utilization of IGF-1 and SirT1 Tg and KO hereditary mice models.

Considering these contemplations, and the set-up job of SirT1 in skeletal muscle cell proliferation and differentiation (Fulco et al., 2003), we foresee that SirT1 agonists and adversaries might be valuable in treating muscle harm. In the underlying periods of muscle damage, SirT1 agonists may help in amplifying the development of the satellite cell pool, and later on, organization of SirT1 rivals may support the differentiation of this extended satellite cell populace.

In both skeletal and heart muscle, quality articulation is managed in a circadian manner (24-hour cycles), and the atomic design of this marvel depends on a mind boggling interpretation criticism circle in which a heterodimeric translation factor, CLOCK/BMAL1, controls the outflow of other clock qualities [such as Bmal1 (otherwise called Arntl), Per2, Dbp, Rora and Cry1]. This atomic circadian clock machine administers the entirety of the physiological rhythms that are available in living creatures, including rest wake cycles and encouraging. Twenty-four-hour rhythms are endogenously produced yet can likewise be entrained by outside signals, for example, light and nourishment accessibility, which follow up on the hypothalamic suprachiasmatic core (SCN) (Crosio et al., 2000). The SCN clock is accepted to set the periods of fringe tissues, for example, skeletal and heart muscle (Lamia et al., 2008). While in the skeletal muscle the circadian clock is essential for action and body weight (Zambon et al., 2003; McDearmon et al., 2006), the cardiovascular clock empowers the heart to foresee natural boosts, guaranteeing a suitable reaction (Esser and Young, 2009). Indeed, diurnal changes in myocardial withdrawals are outstanding, both in mouse models and in people. Clock quality articulation designs are modified in creature models of hypertension, myocardial localized necrosis or ischemia (Esser and Young, 2009), and in people, myocardial dead tissue all the more often happens promptly in the first part of the day and in shift workers (with changed rest wake cycles) (Esser and Young, 2009). Notwithstanding, the reason impact connections of this wonder are not comprehended.

Guideline and Targets of Sirtuins

Sirt1 is broadly communicated in mammalian cells. In spite of the fact that Sirt1 was initially identified as an atomic limiting protein, as of late, its subcellular restriction has been appeared to rely upon cell type. In undeveloped mouse hearts, Sirt1 is exceptionally communicated in the core yet decreases with further organogenesis. The articulation level of Sirt1 in grown-up hearts is about 20% of that in early stage hearts. Sirt3 was initially identified as a mitochondria-limiting protein. Nonetheless, it is additionally found in the core and cytoplasm.

The articulation and movement of Sirt1 are constrained by a few pathophysiological stresses, interpretation elements and cofactors, and post-translational modification. A few administrative elements of Sirt1 have been identified in non-heart cells. Sirt1 is upregulated by E2F1, Forkhead box class O (FoxO) 1, and FoxO3 in mammalian cells (PC cells) and human non-little cell lung carcinoma cells (H1299 cells), while it is curbed by hypermethylated in malignant growth and COOH-terminal restricting protein in fibroblasts. Hu antigen R balances out Sirt1 mRNA(1) in HeLa cells, and a few microRNAs, for example, miR-34a, miR-134, miR-199a, and miR-217, control Sirt1 articulation in neuronal cells and HeLa cells. Cyclin B/cyclin-subordinate kinase 1 and c-Jun NH2-terminal kinase 1 (JNK1) phosphorylate Sirt1, along these lines upgrading its deacetylase action in C2C12 cells and HEK293 cells. Moreover, sumoylation speaks to another significant administrative instrument. Sirt1 deacetylase movement is expanded by sumoylation of Sirt1 at K734, which is curbed by sentrin-specific peptidase 1, in malignant growth cell lines. Sumoylation improves Sirt1 movement during ischemic preconditioning (IPC) in the mouse heart. Dynamic controller of Sirt1 and erased in bosom malignant growth 1 are known as positive and negative controllers in disease cell lines, separately. Moreover, a few caspases stifle the movement of Sirt1 through cleavage and corruption in HeLa cells.

The deacetylase action of Sirt1 is controlled by the accessibility of NAD+. Nicotinamide phosphoribosyl transferase (Nampt) catalyzes the exchange of a phosphoribosyl pyrophosphate to NAM to deliver NAM mononucleotide, subsequently filling in as a rate-constraining protein in the mammalian NAD+ rescue pathway. Late investigations have indicated that Nampt is controlled according to the circadian cadence by clock qualities, including BMAL1 and PER2, by means of Sirt1-intervened deacetylation, which, thus, decidedly directs Sirt1 action in NIH3T3 cells, mouse early stage fibroblasts (MEFs), and hepatocytes. Weight over-burden, supplement starvation, exercise, and intense IPC upregulate Sirt1 in the heart. Nucleocytoplasmic carrying may likewise control the capacity of Sirt1, since Sirt1 has both atomic restriction and atomic fare signals, which are directed by means of phosphorylation by phosphatidylinositol 3-kinase (PI3K) in C2C12 cells. Sirt1 is thought to restrict in both the cytoplasm and the core at benchmark and move to the core considering worry in the heart.

Just a couple of proteins have been exhibited to be legitimately deacetylated and practically directed by Sirt1. These incorporate FoxOs, p53, and poly-adenosine 5'-diphosphate (ADP) - ribose polymerase (PARP) 1. FoxO, a mammalian homolog of Daf16, which is associated with DNA fix, cell cycle, cell demise/endurance, and guideline of responsive oxygen species (ROS), is both decidedly and adversely directed by Sirt1. Sirt1 deacetylates and enacts FoxOs to upregulate articulation of cancer prevention agents, including Mn-superoxide dismutase (MnSOD), catalase, and thioredoxin-1 (Trx1), and antiapoptotic factors, similar to B-cell lymphoma-additional huge (Bcl-xL), in cardiomyocytes. Sirt1 likewise actuates Akt/PI3K flagging, prompting improvement of the cardiovascular hypertrophic reaction.

As portrayed over, the administrative instruments and focuses of Sirt1 have been very much explored. Be that as it may, less is known about those of other sirtuin family proteins. A few investigations have raised the likelihood that sirtuin proteins are managed by a typical pathway and that the sirtuin proteins control each other. AMP-initiated protein kinase (AMPK) expanded articulation of Sirt1, Sirt2, Sirt3, and Sirt6, while Sirt5 mRNA was downregulated, in mouse hepatocytes. Sirt1 can tie and initiate the Sirt6 advertiser, which may amplify the reaction to worry in hepatocytes. As of late, greasy acyl modification of TNF-α was additionally seen as managed by Sirt6 in MEF cells. Sirt6 collaborates with CLOCK/BMAL1 and oversees their chromatin enrollment to circadian quality advertisers in hepatocytes. The jobs of Sirt proteins and their flagging components in the cardiovascular framework are talked about beneath.

Guideline of Energy Metabolism by Sirtuins

The heart is portrayed by high vitality request since its fundamental capacity is to siphon against pulse. Cardiomyocytes assume a focal job in compression of the heart and contain a significant number of mitochondria, which intervene vitality generation. Mitochondria are ATP-delivering organelles that assume a basic job in vitality digestion in the heart. Among the sirtuin family proteins, Sirt1 directs mitochondrial work by deacetylating atomic proteins, though Sirt3 does as such by deacetylating mitochondrial proteins. The heart prevalently utilizes free unsaturated fat as a substrate for adenosine triphosphate (ATP) generation under physiological conditions. In bombing hearts, the favored substrate changes from free unsaturated fat to glucose to create more ATP per particle of oxygen expended. Be that as it may, the propelled bombing heart creates insulin opposition in the myocardium and experiences a decrease in glucose usage, restricting ATP generation.

Peroxisome proliferator-enacted receptor (PPAR)- γ coactivator 1α (PGC-1α), a transcriptional coactivator of atomic receptors, including PPAR-α and estrogen-related receptor (ERR)- α, is an ace controller of digestion and mitochondrial biogenesis. Sirt1 legitimately ties to PGC-1α and deacetylates it in 293T cells and PC12 cells. Sirt1 invigorates the capacity of PGC-1α to coactivate hepatocyte atomic factor 4α, subsequently decidedly controlling gluconeogenic qualities considering pyruvate in hepatic cells. In a similar cell type, Sirt1 likewise improves the capacity of PGC-1α to hinder glycolytic qualities in light of pyruvate. In PC12 cells, wild-type Sirt1, yet not a Sirt1 freak that can't communicate with PGC-1α, adversely manages the transcriptional action of PGC-1α. Accordingly the useful results of PGC-1α deacetylation seem assorted and cell type or interpretation factor subordinate. Moreover, Krishnan et al. Exhibited that Sirt2, yet not Sirt1, influences unsaturated fat oxidation in adipocytes and that knockdown of PGC-1α drops the impact of overexpression of Sirt2 upon unsaturated fat oxidation. In this way the accessibility of other relatives likewise adds to the net impact of sirtuins upon PGC-1α. Fundamental cancellation of Sirt1 in mice prompts the advancement of widened cardiomyopathy, which is joined by mitochondrial brokenness. In any case, Sirt1 is upregulated in the bombing heart and adds to downregulation of qualities engaged with mitochondrial work that are managed by ERRs. Subsequently the impact of Sirt1 upon mitochondrial capacity and digestion in the heart is likewise mind boggling and perhaps portion subordinate.

Overexpression of Sirt1 in pancreatic β-cells upgrades insulin emission in light of glucose and improves glucose digestion by expanding ATP generation by means of concealment of uncoupling protein-2 articulation. Resveratrol, a Sirt1 activator, represses vacuolization, degeneration, and irritation in the heart in an insulin obstruction model. Akt is likewise an objective of Sirt1 in insulin flagging. Akt is acetylated in different tissues, including the heart, under basal conditions, and acetylation of Akt at K14 and K20 stifles Akt action. Deacetylation of Akt by Sirt1 is fundamental for the official of Akt to phosphatidylinositol 3,4,5-trisphosphate (PIP3) in the heart. It ought to be noted, in any case, that one gathering announced that they couldn't distinguish acetylation of Akt in HEK 293T cells. In this way it is conceivable that under some test conditions, the impact of sirtuins upon Akt may not be through direct deacetylation. In cardiomyocytes, overexpression of Sirt1 hindered phenylephrine-actuated downregulation of unsaturated fat oxidation qualities by improving PPAR-α authoritative to the p65 subunit of NF-κB.

THE SIRTFOOD DIET: A LIST WITH THE TOP SIRTFOODS

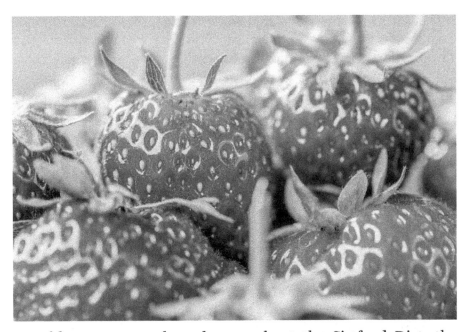

As of late, you may have known about the Sirtfood Diet, the popular eating regimen that guarantees you can lose as much as 7 pounds in 7 days. Established by U.K. sustenance specialists Aidan Goggins and Glen Matten, the Sirtfood Diet vows to invigorate the "thin quality," or the proteins under the SIRT1 quality, to check the impacts of aggravation and weight gain, just as maturing.

The Sirtfood Diet depends on the rule that specific nourishments enact sirtuin, a (profoundly questionable) protein in the body that is claimed to help control digestion and offer cell security to hinder the maturing procedure. Advocates of the eating routine state that eating sirtuin-rich nourishments like green tea, kale, blueberries, salmon, and citrus organic products can give the body a relentless metabolic lift, permitting you to get more fit quick. Such nourishments are likewise stuffed with polyphenols, which are cancer prevention agents that better your skin and heart, says Brooke Alpert, RD and creator of The Diet Detox.

The Sirtfood Diet is part into two stages. The main stage, which keeps going three days, expects you to confine your day by day calorie admission to 1000 calories for every day by drinking three green juices and one sirtfood-rich feast every day. (You increment your dinner check from days 4 to 7 to two suppers and two green juices for every day.) The subsequent stage, the "support" stage, keeps going 14 days and expects you to eat three sirtuin-rich dinners and one green juice for every day.

While the guarantee of the Sirtfood diet is interesting (Adele and Pippa Middleton are apparently fans), and keeping in mind that confining your calories may in reality lead you to shed pounds for the time being, the inquiry remains: is this eating regimen really solid, or is it simply one more senseless (and conceivably hazardous) diet pattern? So far as that is concerned, is it even successful in any case?

First: the Sirtfood diet is as a matter of fact exceptionally prohibitive. In contrast to the Keto or Paleo consumes less calories, which underscore having a decent eating regimen, the Sirtfood diet centers vigorously around tallying calories. It additionally expects you to remove some significant nutritional categories and scale back bits to an extraordinary, if just incidentally. So, for the main week or something like that, you may be passing up lean proteins (hamburger, poultry, and vegetables). While you're despite everything permitted to eat olive oil and pecan (the two of which are wellsprings of sirtuin), the complete day by day carbohydrate content for the main week is incredibly low — under half of what the normal dynamic person needs. It additionally needs other fundamental supplements, like calcium and iron.

It's likewise vague whether sirtuin can really cause weight reduction regardless. Until this point in time, there have been no human investigations absolutely connecting sirtuin-rich nourishments to weight reduction. All things considered, drinking juices that are high in greens and low in sugar for a large portion of the day can without much of a stretch reason transient weight reduction all alone: in case you're getting less calories and remaining hydrated, it bodes well that you'll shed a couple of pounds.

Kristen Smith, MS, RD, LD, a representative for the Academy of Nutrition and Dietetics, backs this up. "It is hard to unravel whether the quick weight reduction guaranteed in the primary seven day stretch of the eating routine is ascribed to the altogether low-calorie diet prescribed or identified with the fat-consuming forces of sirtuin-boosting nourishments," she says.

Fundamentally, "paying little heed to the sirtuin-boosting nourishments, individuals will shed pounds on a 1000-calorie diet," she clarifies.

Alpert concurs. "The creators state that individuals can lose as much as 7 pounds in 7 days yet I wonder the amount of this weight really remains off for longer than one month, if that long," she clarifies.

Regardless of whether you get in shape during that first week, it could be essentially water weight, which implies you may recover it once you begin taking in more calories. Truth be told, you may even put on more weight: as Men's Health has recently announced, when you lose a great deal of weight rapidly, your body's digestion really eases back down, on the grounds that your body is attempting to compensate for its decreased calorie consumption.

Likewise, with any eating regimen, the Sirtfood Diet additionally accompanies its own reactions. While it likely won't do a lot of harm for you to eat so little for the time being, in case you're not used to eating so small during the day, it can cause exhaustion, sickness, weakened mental center, and cerebral pains, says Smith. It can likewise prompt horrendous defecations in case you're not getting enough fiber. Likewise, you may get terrible breath, which can be a reaction of not eating enough.

There is, in any case, one positive: If you eat a great deal of sirtfoods over a continued timeframe, you may see enhancements in heart wellbeing due to the polyphenols in the nourishments you're eating, Smith says. If you keep on eating sirtfoods after you end the eating routine and begin to eat more calories, you'll see the advantages.

The takeaway? While it is probably going to prompt transient weight reduction, the Sirtfood diet is eventually so prohibitive that it's not so much reasonable. Also, if you've at any point had a dietary issue or a confounded association with eating previously, it's ideal to keep away from it out and out, says Alpert.

"I wouldn't prescribe such a low calorie admission for anybody. Extraordinary eating less junk food sets individuals up for horrible dietary patterns and indulging when it's finished," she includes.

All things considered, eating more sirtuin-rich nourishments is without a doubt useful for your wellbeing, so you can undoubtedly bring them into your eating regimen without restricting yourself to each dinner or one squeeze in turn. There's nothing amiss with eating more fish, berries, and verdant greens (particularly in light of the fact that these nourishments are stuffed with fiber and protein) and having a green squeeze that is low in sugar could be an incredible expansion to a previously adjusted eating routine.

At last, you can presumably receive the rewards of the SIRT diet without making a plunge totally. Simply ensure your bits are reasonable and you're getting your calories from a wide assortment of solid sources — no accident eating less junk food or juice fasting important.

The Sirtfood diet has produced a tremendous buzz, just as a top spot on the Amazon smash hit diagrams. With claims that 'sirtfoods' (of which cocoa and red wine are incorporated) "switch on your muscle versus fat's consuming forces, supercharge weight reduction and assist fight with offing ailment", and that the eating regimen could assist you with losing 7lbs in seven days, it's no big surprise individuals are paying heed.

In any case, for the more distrustful among us, it's enticing to hold this eating routine alongside the large number of other "prevailing fashion" weight reduction designs that have gone before it.

Be that as it may, the sirtfood diet professes to be established in science, with more than 100 referenced investigations to back it up, which has made skeptical specialists sit up and give more consideration. So, what precisely are these sirtfoods, and how would they work (if at all...)?

Unfortunately, the Sirtfood diet doesn't permit boundless utilization of red wine and chocolate, in spite of what a few features may have you accept.

As per creators Aidan Goggins and Glen Matten, sirtfoods are a newfound gathering of nourishments, depicted as "especially wealthy in unique supplements that, when we devour them, can actuate a similar thin quality in our body that fasting does". These "thin qualities" are known as sirtuins, a class of proteins that examination has demonstrated to be significant for managing natural pathways which influence our wellbeing and weight.

The writers proceed to depict how "sirtfoods go about as ace controllers of our digestion, most quite having impacts on fat consuming while at the same time expanding muscle and improving cell wellness." The book's best 20 sirtfoods are:

- additional virgin olive oil
- tricks
- red onions
- parsley
- kale
- pecans
- strawberries
- bean stew
- soy items
- cocoa
- green tea
- espresso
- medjool dates
- red chicory
- lovage
- rocket

- celery
- buckwheat
- turmeric
- red wine

What is the Sirtfood diet plan?

The sirtfood diet comprises of two stages. The principal stage, or the "hyper achievement stage", includes three days eating only 1,000 calories per day, comprising of two sirtfood-rich green juices and one sirtfood-rich supper. The following four days incorporate two sirtfood-rich green juices and two sirtfood-rich suppers, at 1,500 calories every day. It is during this "hyper achievement stage" that the creators shellfish members can hope to lose 7lb.

Stage two is the "14-day support stage" during which three adjusted sirtfood-rich dinners and one sirtfood-rich green juice every day is prescribed. After this support stage, center changes to "sirtifying" your eating routine in the long haul, by making nourishment changes to consolidate more sirtfoods into your eating regimen.

The clinical preliminary

The sirtfood diet was tried in a pilot learn at a private exercise center in Chelsea, London. For the examination, 40 people attempted what has now been named the "hyper achievement stage" of the sirtfood diet, more than seven days.

Everything except one member completed the preliminary until the end, and the staying 39 members lost a normal of 7lbs (3.2kg) throughout the week. In addition, bulk was either kept up or expanded. They additionally all detailed inclination and looking more beneficial.

Confinements of this preliminary

This preliminary is generally referred to all through the book as proof of the sirtfood diet's viability. The "lose 7lbs in 7 days" guarantee depends on the discoveries saw right now. In any case, there are a few constraints to this examination I believe merit featuring:

Little example size

Pundits have and will keep on addressing whether it's acceptable logical practice to extrapolate the discoveries from 39 people onto a whole populace. The creators have affirmed that there are discussions in progress for bigger clinical preliminaries to be done, however until these happen this question mark won't leave.

No long haul results

As there was no detailed follow-up to this 7-day preliminary, we don't know whether the members' kept up this weight reduction long haul. Did they set the weight back on when they came back to eating an ordinary eating regimen, without calorie limitation? The book provides tributes on the side of long-haul weight reduction, however there is no information to affirm this.

Test inclination

The preliminary was performed on rec center goers who were at that point sound and practicing routinely. The creators basis behind this was: "On the off chance that we acquired great outcomes with this moderately sound gathering, it would set the base benchmark of what was attainable." I would contend that an increasingly delegate test of the all-inclusive community would have given a more genuine image of how viably the eating regimen could function for the normal individual.

No benchmark group

How might we be sure that the weight reduction watched was because of the impacts of sirtfoods, and not just from calorie limitation? Since a benchmark group wasn't utilized to attempt a similar calorie limitation diet without the incorporation of sirtfoods, we essentially can't reach firm determinations on whether the sirtfoods were a noteworthy contributory factor to the weight reduction.

Weighing up the upsides and downsides of sirtfoods

OK profit by eating more sirtfoods? Unquestionably. In any case, the sirtfood diet feels somewhat like it gains by a large number of individuals' longing to shed pounds quick. Expressions, for example, "turbo-charge your weight reduction" and "lose 7lb in 7 days" propose that the book's essential point is to target people who are searching for a handy solution. This sort of quick weight reduction, by whatever means, is neither solid nor economical.

The creators accentuation it's not just about weight reduction: "To consider it simply as a weight reduction diet is to overlook what's really important. This is an eating regimen that has as a lot to do with health as waistlines," they compose. Removing weight reduction from the condition and setting aside the "hyper achievement stage" of calorie limitation, there is no denying that the guidance to eat more plant nourishments high in fiber, nutrients, cancer prevention agents, phytochemicals and polyphenols will be acceptable wellbeing guidance for everybody.

In any case, while the ebb and flow and developing exploration encompassing sirtfoods is energizing and promising, it is still beginning period. We need bigger scale human investigations, before we can make any firm ends on the job these specific nourishments can have on explicit parts of our wellbeing.

HOW SUPERFOODS PREVENT CANCER

A bowl brimming with splendid green steamed broccoli. You state either "Yum!" - or "Where's the twofold cheeseburger?" But you realize the broccoli is beneficial for you, particularly without softened cheddar. The inquiry is, how acceptable? Furthermore, more to the point, can it - or any food - help forestall illness, for example, malignancy?

The appropriate response is yes - a few foods do show malignancy battling properties; however, nobody is yet ready to state some food can forestall or leave disease speechless. In any case, an assortment of research recommends a general sound diet loaded up with brilliant products of the soil is the way to avoiding coronary illness, diabetes, and conceivably malignancy as well.

Actually, researchers find out about what not to eat - prepared meats, salty foods, sugary beverages, enormous helpings of red meat - than which leafy foods to heap on your plate. Be that as it may, they do realize those foods matter.

A far reaching survey of thousands of concentrates on diet, physical movement, and weight led for the World Cancer Research Fund and the American Institute for Cancer Research highlighted the advantages of eating for the most part foods of plant starting point. Foods, for example, broccoli, berries, and garlic demonstrated the absolute most grounded connections to malignant growth anticipation.

They're low in calories and fat and force pressed with phytochemicals and cell reinforcements that may help diminish your malignant growth chance.

Cell reinforcements, Phytochemicals, and Cancer

You've known about cancer prevention agents, for example, nutrient C, lycopene, and beta-carotene, which are in numerous foods grown from the ground. Studies propose that individuals who eat dinners that are wealthy in leafy foods have a lower danger of malignant growth. An assortment of synthetic concoctions from plants known as phytochemicals likewise appear to shield cells from destructive mixes in food and in the earth, just as forestall cell harm and transformations, says Jed W. Fahey, ScD, MS, an associate teacher at Johns Hopkins Bloomberg School of Public Health and its School of Medicine who contemplates how cruciferous vegetables help secure against malady.

A diet that could avoid malignancy truly doesn't appear to be that unique from the solid foods you ought to eat at any rate, says Wendy Demark-Wahnefried, PhD, RD,associate chief for Cancer Prevention and Control at the University of Alabama's Comprehensive Cancer Center. That implies a lot of leafy foods, just as entire grains and lean meat or fish.

What's more, weight matters as well. Keep the scale at a solid number and shed a few pounds if required. Being overweight or hefty builds your danger of creating esophageal malignancy, postmenopausal bosom disease, colorectal disease, endometrial disease, ovarian disease, and others.

So, what foods would it be a good idea for you to stack up on to give your body the most obvious opportunity with regards to avoiding disease? WebMD examined investigate, at times clashing, to coax out certain foods you'll need to eat a lot of, beginning at this moment.

A bowl brimming with brilliant green steamed broccoli. You state either "Yum!" - or "Where's the twofold cheeseburger?" But you realize the broccoli is beneficial for you, particularly without liquefied cheddar. The inquiry is, how acceptable? What's more, more to the point, can it - or any food - help forestall ailment, for example, malignancy?

The appropriate response is yes - a few foods do show malignant growth battling properties; however, nobody is yet ready to state some food can forestall or leave disease speechless. All things considered, an assortment of research recommends a general sound diet loaded up with brilliant products of the soil is the way to avoiding coronary illness, diabetes, and conceivably disease as well.

Truth be told, researchers find out about what not to eat - prepared meats, salty foods, sugary beverages, gigantic helpings of red meat - than which leafy foods to heap on your plate. In any case, they do realize those foods matter.

A complete audit of thousands of concentrates on diet, physical movement, and weight directed for the World Cancer Research Fund and the American Institute for Cancer Research highlighted the advantages of eating for the most part foods of plant starting point. Foods, for example, broccoli, berries, and garlic indicated the absolute most grounded connections to disease avoidance.

They're low in calories and fat and force pressed with phytochemicals and cell reinforcements that may help lessen your malignant growth chance.

From ensuring your vision to helping in weight loss and forestalling diabetes, the foods on this rundown all contain various medical advantages. However, the one thing that they all share for all intents and purpose – they are malignant growth battling superfoods.

Broccoli

Broccoli, kale, asparagus, Brussels sprouts and cauliflower are for the most part hostile to malignant growth superfoods, Connie Rogers, Certified Integrative Nutritional Holistic Health Coach, says. "Cruciferous vegetables contain sulforophane, which has against disease properties."

Nutrient D Rich Foods

Nutrient D rich foods including natural shiitake mushrooms, sweet potatoes, sunflower sprouts, and fenugreek have against malignant growth properties, Rogers says. "As people we blossom with sun presentation for cerebrum and entire body wellbeing. Moreover, ingesting natural nutrient D rich foods has strong enemy of malignant growth properties. Stay away from fortified or enhanced foods that can contain hurtful synthetics."

Matured Foods

"These foods incorporate natural crude sauerkraut or matured crude carrots," Rogers says. "Improved gut microbiome can be malignant growth deterrent. Probiotic defensive microbes decrease the degree of cancer-causing action."

Wheatgrass

Wheatgrass is viewed as a detoxifying therapeutic herb. "Medical advantages incorporate improving red platelet tally and killing ecological poisons inside the body," Rogers says. "Wheatgrass additionally shows benefits in malignant growth anticipation. You can utilize wheatgrass by squeezing it day by day in 2oz shots."

Parsley

"Parsley is a superfood used to treat a wide assortment of conditions and help forestall oxidative pressure illnesses, for example, malignancy," Rogers says. "Quercetin is a plant shade found in green verdant herbs, for example, parsley and leafy foods, for example, berries and broccoli. It contains cancer prevention agents, calming, hostile to viral and against malignant growth properties, and battles free extreme harm." Quercetin can hinder the development of disease cells with the capacity to go about as chemo preventers, she includes.

DIET PLAN TO LOSE 7LBS IN 7 DAYS

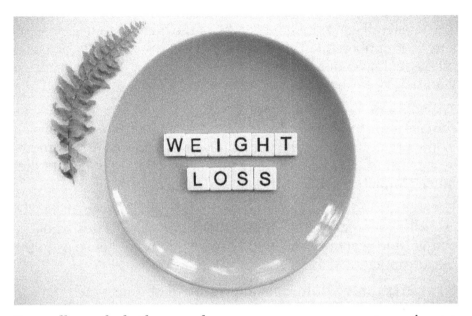

Regardless of whether you have an uncommon event coming up or are streaming off to a sea shore occasion one week from now, we have the ideal good dieting intend to assist you with shedding pounds rapidly.

So, would you be able to get in shape in seven days? With the multi week diet plan, you could lose as much as seven pounds in seven days.

Getting trim can be precarious and attempting to get in shape quick can be significantly increasingly difficult. Over and over again, we promise to hit the rec center each morning and subsist on only one low-cal feast every day, just to wind up falling flat and gorging on cake and chocolate on day two. That is on the grounds that prevailing fashion diets can be extraordinarily prohibitive and often leave us feeling ravenous and unsatisfied – also ailing in vitality.

No more! With the multi week diet plan, you can get in shape quick and feel extraordinary in only seven days – without starving yourself in route. Win big or bust diets set you up for disappointment, however the multi week diet plan permits you to eat three full suppers for each day, including bunches of solid foods grown from the ground, in addition to eating in the middle of dinners.

You'll feel full and fulfilled, because of the high protein admission and a lot of fiber-filled vegetables and natural products. Sugar is off the menu yet don't stress, you're despite everything permitted your day by day espresso or tea fix – simply ensure its decaf!

There are no contrivances to the multi week diet, simply savvy counsel and simple to-adhere to guidelines. The weight loss plan is low in fat, low in carbs, yet high in bravo foods. Furthermore, best of all, dinners can be put together quick, making the diet much simpler to adhere to!

If you're wanting to shift the pounds in only seven days, it's critical to shoulder at the top of the priority list that it won't be simple, and that you'll need to keep up a limited diet so as to see the advantages.

So as to get more fit in such a little space of time, you'll have to keep your carbohydrate content low, while as yet keeping up a solid diet plan that will keep you fulfilled – as, obviously, you're bound to need the terrible stuff if you aren't!

The most effective method to get in shape in seven days: The supper plans

Regardless of whether you have a unique event coming up or are flying off to a sea shore occasion one week from now, we have the ideal good dieting intend to assist you with shedding pounds quick. Truth be told, with the multi week diet plan, you could lose as much as seven pounds in seven days!

Getting thinner can be difficult and attempting to shed pounds quick can feel practically unthinkable. Again, and again, we promise to hit the exercise center each morning and attempt to subsist on only one low-cal supper every day, just to wind up falling flat and gorging on cake and chocolate on day two.

That is on the grounds that prevailing fashion diets can be extraordinarily prohibitive and often leave us feeling ravenous and unsatisfied – also ailing in vitality. No more! With the multi week diet plan, you can get in shape and feel extraordinary in only seven days – without starving yourself in route.

There are no tricks to the multi week diet, simply savvy counsel and simple to-adhere to directions. The weight loss plan is low in fat, low in carbs however high in bravo foods. Best of all, dinners can be put together quick, making the diet significantly simpler to adhere to!

Win big or bust diets set you up for disappointment. Be that as it may, the multi week diet plan permits you to eat three full suppers for each day, including loads of sound products of the soil, in addition to nibbling in the middle of dinners. You'll feel full and fulfilled, on account of the high protein admission and a lot of nutritious foods. Sugar is off the menu however don't stress, you're despite everything permitted your day by day espresso or tea fix – simply ensure it's decaf!

Down beneath is a rundown of food things and tips I utilized for results. I am as of now despite everything dieting and working out. I would incline toward the term lifestyle change. Recall if you return to your old propensities you will in the long run recover the weight. This ought to be a lifestyle change. That is all! Actually, I see myself down the line being a veggie lover. NO LIE! Yet, then again I'm poor ehehehe.

Appropriately note I am not a nutritionist or dietician or master of any kind. Endeavoring a diet and practicing plan may require endorsement from your primary care physician, particularly if you have any hidden ailments. I can reveal to you that I have done this specific diet and have gotten results just by actualizing this low carb, low sugar decisions. This can be proceeded on a more extended premise and doesn't really implies a momentary handy solution. This diet won't starve you, by eating these foods you ought to be fulfilled and support.

If you might want to do the diet long haul, I will recommend including snacks in your diet. For a convenient solution stay away from the bites and do quality preparing exercise in any event three times each week.

Right off the bat, let me start with the DO'S and the DON'TS

- Maintain a strategic distance from Condiments
- Eat less carbs and increasingly lean protein
- Eat More Veggies (Whole Food)
- Try not to drink your calories. Drink ONLY WATER or GREEN TEA
- Maintain a strategic distance from Processed Foods
- Eat just suppers. Nibble ONLY if didn't eat enough calorie.
- Tally your Calories
- Take your enhancements
- Protein Shakes are extraordinary for dinner substitutions
- Keep nibble beneath 150 calories
- Try not to Skip Meals
- Drink heaps of water for the duration of the day (This straightforwardness hunger)

If you have a functioning activity attempt to expand your calorie consumption by the most 300 calories, by including snacks.

The very beginning

DAY ONE

- **Breakfast**: Oatmeal and Watermelon. Drink cup of Green Tea
- **Lunch**: Tuna Sandwich enveloped by lettuce. Drink Glass of water

- **Supper**: Bake/Roast Chicken with Spinach with broccoli

DAY TWO

- **Breakfast**: Boiled or Scrambled eggs/No margarine with 1 cut of toast. Drink Cup Green Tea
- **Lunch**: Chicken Salad with No cream dressing
- **Supper**: Salmon and Asparagus or Green Beans

DAY THREE

- **Breakfast**: 2 Piece of Waffles and a Fruit No syrup. Drink Cup Green Tea
- **Lunch**: Sandwich (Whole Grain Bread) of Choice (Lean Meat) (No Fry)
- **Supper**: Roast Beef with 1/2 cup of Jasmine Rice and Veggies as an afterthought

DAY FOUR

- **Breakfast**: Boiled or Scrambled eggs/No margarine with 1 cut of toast. Drink Cup Green Tea
- **Lunch**: Chicken Salad with No cream dressing
- **Supper**: Salmon/Shrimp and Veggies

DAY FIVE

- **Breakfast**: Oatmeal and a natural product. Drink a cup green tea.
- **Lunch**: Protein Shake
- **Supper**: Take Out (make sure to eat clean)

DAY SIX

- **Breakfast**: Choose your Breakfast

- **Lunch**: Salad of Choice with a Protein
- **Supper**: Bake/Roast Chicken with 1/2 of Sweet potato and Veggies

DAY SEVEN

- **Breakfast**: Boiled or Scrambled eggs/No spread with 1 cut of toast. Drink Cup Green Tea
- **Lunch**: Protein Shake or Chicken Salad
- **Supper**: Choice of lean Protein, 1/2 cup of rice and Veggies

Nibble Options (Only if required)

- Low Fat Yogurt
- Carrots
- Bunch of Peanuts or Almond
- Natural products (Melon, Orange, Cantaloupe, Grapes, Pineapple, Kiwi, Banana any Berry Fruit)

By Implementing this diet, plan I am certain you will get in shape. I have been doing this for some time, and I am getting in shape, and I feel incredible. In addition to the fact that I feel incredible, however I am not constantly eager. I will update you as often as possible and obviously, toward the finish of excursion show my before and after pictures.

Try not to attempt to put off getting thinner It isn't justified, despite any potential benefits, tomorrow may simply be another tomorrow. If you have any inquiries simply let me know.

SIRTFOOD RECIPES

This supper plan contains fixings wealthy in aggravates that have been appeared to initiate sirtuins. Sirtuins effectsly affect wellbeing that may assist with fighting off malady and lengthen lifespan. It additionally contains fixings wealthy in niacin, a forerunner to NAD+ which is expected to initiate sirtuins. If it's not too much trouble read the sirt foods bulletin for more data on sirtuins and their belongings. Dinners with a * have a formula in the Sirt Foods formula area.

WEEK 1

MONDAY

Breakfast: Chia breakfast bowl – Soak 2 tbsp of chia protein powder in ½ cup of oat or almond milk for 20 minutes. Mix in blueberries and hacked nuts and serve.

Bite: An apple

Lunch: Almond spread and horse feed wraps*

Bite: Carrot sticks with dark olive tapenade

Supper: Buckwheat and nut loaf* with green serving of mixed greens and olive oil and lemon dressing

TUESDAY

Breakfast: Tofu Berry Smoothie – Blend together 100g of luxurious tofu with ½ cup of strawberries and a tsp of cacao powder. Sprinkle with hulled hemp seeds.

Tidbit: A pear

Lunch: Buckwheat and nut portion from yesterday

Bite: Celery sticks with almond margarine

Supper: Quinoa, edamame and pomegranate seed pilaf*

WEDNESDAY

Breakfast: Rye toast with pumpkin seed spread

Bite: a kiwi natural product

Lunch: Quinoa and edamame bean pilaf from yesterday

Bite: A couple of olives

Supper: Sweet Potato and Salmon Patties* with watercress and rocket serving of mixed greens

THURSDAY

Breakfast: Normal yogurt with berries and blackcurrants

Tidbit: A pink grapefruit

Lunch: Sweet Potato and Salmon Patties from yesterday

Tidbit: Cucumber sticks with hummus

Supper: Moong dahl* with red rice

FRIDAY

Breakfast: Sugar free muesli with common soya yogurt

Bite: A couple of dried figs

Lunch: Moong dahl and rice from yesterday

Tidbit: A couple of walnut nuts and a carrot

Supper: Dill simmered mackerel with tomatoes and steamed vegetables*

SATURDAY

Breakfast: Bubbled natural eggs with toasted rye bread

Tidbit: A cup of blueberries

Lunch: Crude carrot and almond loaf* with green serving of mixed greens

Tidbit: Celery sticks with dark olive tapenade

Supper: Buckwheat Bean and Tomato Risotto*

SUNDAY

Breakfast: Regular yogurt with berries, blackcurrants and nuts

Tidbit: Oat cakes with almond margarine

Lunch: Buckwheat bean and tomato risotto from yesterday

Tidbit: ½ an avocado

Supper: Crude carrot and almond portion from yesterday with grow serving of mixed greens

WEEK 2

MONDAY

Breakfast: Sugar free muesli with oat milk

Bite: A grapefruit

Lunch: Flavorful seed truffles* with rocket and watercress

Bite: ½ an avocado

Supper: Trout with cooked vegetables*

TUESDAY

Breakfast: Seed and Berry Breakfast Bowl – Put 1 tbsp pumpkin seed protein powder and 1 tbsp of hemp seed protein powder in a bowl with some nut milk. Include berries and cleaved nuts.

Bite: A pear

Lunch: Almond spread and horse feed wraps*

Bite: Flavorful seed truffles from yesterday

Supper: Courgette Tortilla* with green plate of mixed greens and olive oil and lemon dressing

WEDNESDAY

Breakfast: Porridge with tahini

Bite: A kiwi natural product

Lunch: Courgette tortilla from yesterday

Bite: Celery sticks with hummus

Supper: Polenta bake* with steamed kale and broccoli

THURSDAY

Breakfast: Chia berry smoothie – mix ½ an avocado with 1 tbsp chia protein powder and a cup of berries. Add fluid to make wanted consistency.

Bite: An apple

Lunch: Polenta heat from yesterday

Tidbit: Buckwheat saltines with pumpkin seed margarine

Supper: Butterbean and vegetable korma* with red rice

FRIDAY

Breakfast: Sugar free muesli with regular yogurt

Tidbit: An enthusiasm organic product

Lunch: Butterbean and vegetable korma from yesterday

Tidbit: A couple of olives

Supper: Heated salmon with sautéed vegetables*

SATURDAY

Breakfast: Buckwheat pancakes* with lemon juice, berries and yogurt

Tidbit: vegetable juice – juice celery, beetroot, kale and ginger

Lunch: Pea, miso and mint soup* with ground carrot serving of mixed greens

Tidbit: A cupful of raspberries

Supper: Buckwheat noodles with vegetarian pesto and steamed green vegetables

SUNDAY

Breakfast: Normal yogurt with blueberries and cacao nibs

Tidbit: A cup of red grapes

Lunch: Lemon paprika chicken with vegetables*

Tidbit: A couple of Brazil nuts

Supper: Pea, miso and mint soup from yesterday with ground beetroot plate of mixed greens

WEEK 3

MONDAY

Breakfast: Rye toast with nutty spread

Bite: a bunch of goji berries

Lunch: lemon paprika chicken with vegetables from yesterday

Bite: A couple of almonds

Supper: Tofu pan sear

TUESDAY

Breakfast: Banana berry cacao smoothie – consolidate 1 banana, 1 cup of berries and a tbsp of cacao powder in a blender. Include fluid if wanted.

Bite: Buckwheat wafers with hazelnut margarine

Lunch: Tofu pan sear from yesterday

Tidbit: Carrot sticks with hummus

Supper: Sweet potato and salmon patties* with rocket and tomato serving of mixed greens

WEDNESDAY

Breakfast: Sugar free muesli with oat milk

Tidbit: A pink grapefruit

Lunch: Sweet potato and salmon patties from yesterday

Tidbit: A couple of almonds

Supper: Buckwheat Noodle and Green Bean Soup*

THURSDAY

Breakfast: Mix a ready avocado with a tablespoon of cacao powder and some normal soya or sheep's yogurt.

Tidbit: A kiwi organic product

Lunch: Buckwheat Noodle and Green Bean Soup from yesterday

Tidbit: A cup of blueberries

Supper: Polenta bake* with steamed broccoli and kale

FRIDAY

Breakfast: Normal yogurt with toasted seeds

Tidbit: Apple cuts with nutty spread

Lunch: Polenta heat from yesterday

Tidbit: Carrot sticks with dark olive tapenade

Supper: Dill broiled mackerel with tomatoes and steamed vegetables*

SATURDAY

Breakfast: Consolidate buckwheat chips with a determination of slashed nuts and seeds and some rice or oat milk.

Bite: A pear

Lunch: Avocado and Cannellini Mash Tacos*

Bite: A bunch of goji berries and pumpkin seeds

Supper: Quinoa, edamame and pomegranate seed pilaf*

SUNDAY

Breakfast: Mushroom omelet

Bite: Carrot, kale, apple and ginger juice

Lunch: Quinoa, edamame and pomegranate seed pilaf from yesterday

Bite: A couple of olives

Supper: Green Bean, Tomato and Almond Stir Fry*

This has been my go-to breakfast for the past couple weeks and it's delightful. Indeed, I'm still on the SIRTfood method for eating – I love it, I have a great deal of vitality and I've kept the weight off that I lost at first. Anyway, why change something if it's not broken right? If you can't deal with the testiness of the pepper, ensure you deseed it before tossing it in the skillet or you may be overwhelmed.

BREAKFAST

SirtFood Mushroom Scramble Eggs

Fixings

- ❖ 2 eggs
- ❖ 1 tsp ground turmeric
- ❖ 1 tsp gentle curry powder
- ❖ 20g kale, generally hacked
- ❖ 1 tsp additional virgin olive oil
- ❖ ½ 10,000 foot stew, daintily cut
- ❖ bunch of catch mushrooms, daintily cut
- ❖ 5g parsley, finely hacked
- ❖ *optional* Add a seed blend as a topper and some Rooster Sauce for season

Directions:

Blend the turmeric and curry powder and include a little water until you have accomplished a light glue.

Steam the kale for 2–3 minutes.

Warmth the oil in a griddle over a medium warmth and fry the bean stew and mushrooms for 2–3 minutes until they have begun to dark colored and soften.

Include the eggs and zest glue and cook over a medium warmth then add the kale and keep on cooking over a medium warmth for a further moment. At long last, include the parsley, blend well and serve.

POWER JUICE AND COCKTAILS

Fixings

- ❖ 75 g Kale (2 huge bunches)
- ❖ 30 g Rocket (1 huge bunch)
- ❖ 5 g Flat-leaf parsley (exceptionally little bunch)
- ❖ 5 g Lovage leaves, discretionary (exceptionally little bunch)
- ❖ 150 g Celery, 2-3 sticks including leaves
- ❖ 1/2 Medium green apple (discretionary; can be supplanted by the ginger)
- ❖ Juice of 1/2 a lemon
- ❖ 1/2 tsp. Matcha powder

Directions

Blend the greens (kale, rocket, parsley and lovage) together, then squeeze them. We discover juicers can truly differ in their productivity at squeezing verdant vegetables, and you may need to re-juice the leftovers before proceeding onward to different fixings. The objective is to wind up with about 50ml of juice from the greens.

Presently squeeze the celery and apple or ginger or both.

You can strip the lemon and put it through the juicer too, yet we think that it's a lot simpler to just crush the lemon by hand into the juice. By this stage, you ought to have around 250ml of juice altogether, maybe somewhat more.

It is just when the juice is made and prepared to serve that you include the matcha. Pour a modest quantity of the juice into a glass, then include the matcha and mix vigor- ously with a fork or teaspoon. We use matcha just in the initial two beverages of the day as it contains moderate measures of caffeine (a similar substance as a typical cup of tea). For individuals not accustomed to it, it might keep them wakeful if alcoholic late.

Once the matcha has broken down, include the rest of the juice. Give it a last mix and your juice is prepared to drink; don't hesitate to top it up with plain water, according to taste.

You can either make every juice without any preparation as and when you need it, or you can make up the entirety of your juices for the day in one cluster in the first part of the day, and refrigerate until required, with no loss of power. Truth be told, examine focuses to the gainful sirtuin-activating polyphenols going on for as long as three days before levels begin to drop, so if you're lacking in time, it's flawlessly fine to make your juices ahead of time, guaranteeing you keep them chilled and away from light.

SIMPLE SNACKS

1. Green tea

1 cup (200ml) • 1 of your SIRT 5 per day • 0 calories

Never at any point, think little of the solid SIRT support that some green tea can give you. Have the same number of cups as you can every day – we prescribe in any event two cups. Not just that, the SIRTs in green tea are aggregate so you can find a good pace parts of SIRTs every day if you have four cups of green tea or more.

2. Red grapes

10 grapes • 1 of your SIRT 5 per day • 30 calories

One more of the exceptionally simple Sirtfood snacks and a low-calorie approach to get one of your SIRT parcels. Keep a punnet or two in the refrigerator and have a bunch at breakfast or lunch or even both!

3. Apples

1 apple • 1 of your SIRT 5 per day • 47 calories

An apple daily truly keeps the specialist away. Reach for an apple as one of your after-lunch simple Sirtfood snacks. It will assist keep with sugaring longings under control as well.

4. Cocoa

2 tsp/10g cocoa • 1 of your SIRT 5 every day • 33 calories

Have a go at making a chocolate shot with 2 tsp cocoa. 1 tsp sugar and 30ml milk. Combine the cocoa and sugar with a touch of bubbling water from the pot to make a smooth glue. Mix in the milk. A (nearly) moment chocolate hit with just 68 calories.

5. Olives

6 huge dark or green olives • 1 of your SIRT 5 every day • 75 calories

A flexible and simple Sirtfood nibble toward the evening or a pre-supper treat. Serve at room temperature to get a fuller flavor.

6. Blackberries

15 blackberries • 1 of your SIRT 5 every day • 32 calories

One more of the simple Sirtfood tidbits to keep in your cooler. Additionally, extraordinary as a solidified treat.

7. Dark chocolate 85%

6 squares/20g chocolate • 1 of your SIRT 5 every day • 125 calories

Get your chocolate hit here! If you lean toward 70% dull chocolate, you'll need 9 squares/30g. which will be 180 calories.

8. Pomegranate seeds

50g/a large portion of a little pack • 1 of your SIRT 5 per day • 50 calories

Simple to get while in a hurry, pomegranate seeds sneak up all of a sudden and you just need a large portion of a 100g pack to get one of your SIRT partitions.

9. Blueberries

25 blueberries (80g) • 1 of your sirt 5 every day • 36 cals

One enormous bunch of blueberries can likewise be one of your simple Sirtfood snacks

Are there any advantageous Sirtfood snacks? Eating feels like a word stacked with negative undertones, conjuring pictures of sugar-stacked confectionary or salt-loaded appetizing items. The food business knows very well indeed our soft spot for everything sweet, salty and high in fat, and schemes to guarantee they are never a long way from eyeshot as we approach our day by day lives, an ever-present enticement.

Regardless of whether you're ready for settling on a more beneficial decision, it's a long way from obvious, when tidbits advertised as 'all common' or with 'no additional sugar' can once in a while be as high in sugars as their shoddy nourishment partners. The main difference being that the sugars happen inside the normally sweet fixings they use as opposed to the demonstration of including sugar itself. Investigate the mark and you'll before long observe that there can be astounding measures of sugar concealed away in purported solid snacks as nectar, maple syrup, agave, dried natural products (yet read on for increasingly about dates later, etc. The end result is the equivalent – it's as yet a high sugar nibble, only a ton increasingly costly.

Thus, tidbits can often wind up cheapening the wholesome nature of the diet, when they could really be an opportunity to decidedly upgrade it. So, what would it be a good idea for us to nibble on? Is it true that they are any Sirtfood snacks? There are some of the best 20 Sirtfoods that can be utilized as the reason for solid Sirtfood snacks.

Nuts must be the prototype nutritious nibble food, stacked with 'great' unsaturated fats, plant protein, fiber, and an abundance of nutrients, minerals, and polyphenols. With accreditations like that it's no big surprise that consistently eating nuts slices the danger of coronary illness. What's more, in complete differentiation to other high fat tidbits, consistently eating nuts is connected to having a slimmer waistline, likely because of their amazing satisfying impact. Pecans, specifically are an incredible sirtuin-enacting food and a pleasant Sirtfood nibble. Best of all nuts are tote and office work area agreeable.

Next in the nibbling stakes, and the ideal accomplice to nuts, is dim chocolate (preferably with an 80-85% cocoa content). This is another best 20 Sirtfood. Cocoa contains incredible normally happening plant mixes, known as flavanols, which are presently the subject of escalated scientific research for their medical advantages, particularly for cardiovascular wellbeing. Truth be told, consolidate a couple of squares of dim chocolate with a little bunch of nuts and you have pretty much the most cardio-defensive bite going. Furthermore, much the same as nuts, this is a tidbit that will easily space in a purse or fold

As a feature of the Sirtfood Diet these Dark Chocolate Bites are a firm family most loved as one of the most delightful Sirtfood snacks. It consolidates a large group of wellbeing advancing polyphenols into a liberal treat. While Medjool dates are normally high in sugar (an amazing 66%!), eaten with some restraint they really have no observable glucose raising impacts and are really connected to having less diabetes and coronary illness, on account of their remarkable polyphenol content. This makes them probably the most advantageous alternative for conjuring up a sweet treat.

Dim Chocolate Bits Recipe-Sirtfood Snack

Makes 15–20 nibbles sirtfood snacks

- ❖ 120g pecans
- ❖ 30g dull chocolate (85 percent cocoa solids), broken into pieces; or cocoa nibs
- ❖ 250g Medjool dates, pitted

- ❖ 1 tbsp cocoa powder
- ❖ 1 tbsp ground turmeric
- ❖ 1 tbsp additional virgin olive oil
- ❖ the scratched seeds of 1 vanilla unit or 1 tsp vanilla concentrate
- ❖ 1–2 tbsp water

Spot the pecans and chocolate in a food processor and procedure until you have a fine powder.

Include the various fixings aside from the water and mix until the blend frames a ball. You might possibly need to include the water depending the consistency of the blend – you don't need it to be excessively clingy.

Utilizing your hands, structure the blend into reduced down balls and refrigerate in a hermetically sealed compartment for at any rate 1 hour before eating them. You could move a portion of the balls in some more cocoa or dried up coconut to accomplish a different completion if you like. They will keep for as long as multi week in your ice chest.

CAKES AND BAKING

In the same way as other individuals, Gina Homolka began putting on weight in her twenties—despite the fact that she had a feeling that she was eating very similar things she generally had been. Joining Weight Watchers helped, yet she despite everything battled to discover sound foods that she really delighted in eating. "Certainly, there were a lot of supposed 'diet' plans out there, however a considerable lot of them utilized handled foods or they tated, well, diet-y," she says.

Maple–Raisin Bread Pudding

I've constantly discovered bread pudding entirely difficult to oppose, particularly when it's despite everything warm from the broiler and beat with a bit of whipped cream. Yet, how would you make a pastry that depends on bread and eggs somewhat better or you? I swapped the white bread for entire wheat French bread, swapped the cream for sans fat milk, and cut back on the eggs. To improve it, I like to go regular, utilizing unadulterated maple syrup and raisins rather than refined sugar. In any case, generally significant, I hold parcels within proper limits by preparing them in singular ramekins, so I don't "incidentally" have too much.

- ❖ 2 cups (2 ½ oz) entire wheat French bread, hulls expelled, cut into ½-inch shapes
- ❖ 1 cup without fat milk
- ❖ ¼ cup unadulterated maple syrup
- ❖ 2 ½ tsp unadulterated vanilla concentrate
- ❖ 2 huge eggs
- ❖ ⅓ cup raisins
- ❖ Cooking splash or oil sir

1. Preheat the stove to 350°F.

2. Orchestrate the bread 3D shapes in a solitary layer on a heating sheet. Heat until brilliant, 5 to 6 minutes, mixing part of the way through the cooking time. Let cool.

3. In a medium bowl, whisk together the milk, 3 Tbsp of the maple syrup, vanilla, and eggs. Mix in the raisins. Overlay in the toasted bread 3D shapes. Cover and refrigerate for at any rate 30 minutes or as long as 4 hours.

4. Preheat the stove to 325°F. Splash 4 (5-oz) ramekins with oil. Partition the bread blend similarly among the readied ramekins. Put the ramekins in a 8 × 8-inch heating container, and add 1 inch high temp water to the skillet.

5. Heat until set, 45 to 50 minutes. Sprinkle with outstanding tablespoon of maple syrup. Serve warm.

Makes 4 ramekins. Per ramekin: 172 calories, 0.5 g fat (0 g soaked), 35 g carbs, 143 mg sodium, 23 g sugar, 1 g fiber, 6 g protein.

Twofold Chocolate Chunk Walnut Cookies

I've done some insane, capricious things in preparing, however utilizing avocados instead of margarine may simply be the craziest. In all honesty, it works! For these chewy treats made with lumps of chocolate and pecans in each nibble, I use positively no spread. They taste too great to ever be light—and you can't identify the flavor of avocados by any means. I tried these out on numerous clueless grown-ups, youngsters, and teenagers, and everybody cherished them. Karina, my school age girl, was a definitive test—she's a genuine chocoholic. She believes they're really marvelous!

❖ Cooking shower or oil (discretionary)

❖ 1/2 cup crude sugar

❖ 1/3 cup unloaded dim darker sugar

❖ 1/4 cup pounded avocado

❖ 1 Tbsp unsweetened fruit purée

❖ 1 enormous egg white

❖ 1 tsp unadulterated vanilla concentrate

❖ 1/2 cup (65 grams) white entire wheat unbleached flour (I prescribe King Arthur)

❖ 1/3 cup (50 grams) universally handy flour

❖ 1/3 cup unsweetened cocoa powder (I use Trader Joe's)

❖ 1/4 tsp heating pop

❖ 1/8 tsp fit salt

❖ 1/3 cup semisweet chocolate lumps

❖ 1/2 cup finely slashed pecans

1. Preheat the broiler to 350°F. Line 2 standard preparing sheets with silicone heating mats, (for example, Silpats) or softly shower nonstick preparing sheets with oil.

2. In an enormous bowl, utilizing an electric hand blender, whisk together the sugars, avocado, fruit purée, egg white, and vanilla until the sugar breaks up, around 2 to 3 minutes.

3. In a different enormous bowl, whisk together the flours, cocoa powder, preparing pop, and salt. Crease in the dry fixings with a spatula in two increments. Utilizing a spatula, overlap in the chocolate lumps and pecans. The mixture will be extremely clingy. Spread the bowl with saran wrap and refrigerate 15 minutes. 3 g fiber, 3 g protein.

Pumpkin-Obsessed Vanilla-Glazed Scones

These light and soft buttermilk scones—made with pumpkin puree, fall flavors, and a vanilla bean coat—will heat up your home and fill it with an inebriating aroma that no extravagant flame can verge on recreating. I've helped these up generously by utilizing low-fat buttermilk rather than cream and supplanting some margarine with pumpkin puree. They taste similarly comparable to any scone you would purchase in an extravagant coffeehouse—with a large portion of the calories.

For the scones:

- ❖ Cooking shower or oil
- ❖ ½ cup cold low-fat 1% buttermilk
- ❖ 1 enormous egg
- ❖ 1 tsp unadulterated vanilla concentrate
- ❖ 5 Tbsp canned unsweetened pumpkin puree
- ❖ ¼ cup pressed dull dark colored sugar
- ❖ 1 vanilla bean
- ❖ 1 cup white entire wheat flour (I prescribe King Arthur)
- ❖ 1 cup unbleached universally handy flour, in addition to additional for the work surface
- ❖ 1 Tbsp heating powder
- ❖ 2 tsp pumpkin pie zest

- ❖ 1⁄4 tsp ground nutmeg
- ❖ 1⁄4 tsp ground cinnamon
- ❖ 1⁄2 tsp fit salt
- ❖ 3 Tbsp freezing spread, cut into little pieces

For the coating:

- ❖ 2 Tbsp cold without fat milk
- ❖ 1 cup powdered sugar, sifted

1. Preheat the stove to 375°F. Shower a heating sheet with oil.

2. For the scones: In a medium bowl, whisk together the buttermilk, egg, vanilla, pumpkin puree, and dark colored sugar. Utilizing the tip of a sharp knife, cut along the length of the vanilla bean to part it open. Scratch half of the seeds into the bowl and whisk well; hold the rest of the seeds for the coating.

3. In a huge bowl, whisk together the flours, preparing powder, pumpkin pie zest, nutmeg, cinnamon, and salt. Utilizing a baked good blender or 2 blades, cut in the chilled spread until the blend takes after coarse feast. Include the buttermilk blend, and mix until simply wet. Turn the batter out onto a floured work surface, and manipulate softly multiple times with floured hands. Move the mixture to the preparing sheet, and shape it into a 9-inch circuitous 3⁄4 inch thick. Utilizing a knife, cut the mixture entirely through into 12 wedges.

4. Prepare until brilliant darker, 18 to 20 minutes. Move to a wire rack, and let cool for around 10 minutes before coating.

5. For the coating: Meanwhile, in a medium bowl, whisk together the rest of the seeds from the vanilla bean and the milk. In another medium bowl, include the powdered sugar. Utilizing a spatula, blend in the milk and consolidate well until it is blended through and structures a thick coating.

6. Put the scones on material or wax paper, and shower the vanilla coating over the scones utilizing a spoon. On the other hand, you can plunge the highest points of the scones into the coating and afterward let them sit on the paper to solidify.

7. Serve warm. Remains can be put away in water/air proof holders for as long as 2 days.

Tip: For impeccable scones, be mindful so as not to overwork the mixture, and be certain your margarine is all around chilled. I generally keep a stick of margarine in the cooler only for making scones.

Makes 12 scones. Per scone: 172 calories, 4 g fat (2 g immersed), 32 g carbs, 214 mg sodium, 15 g sugar, 2 g fiber, 4 g protein.

EXCERCISING

Joining The Sirtfood Diet and exercise

With 52% of Americans admitting that they think that its simpler to do their charges than to see how to eat steadily, it's fundamental to present a type of eating that turns into a lifestyle as opposed to a coincidental prevailing fashion diet. For a few of us it may not be that difficult to get thinner or hold a solid weight, however the Sirtfood diet can help the individuals who are battling. Be that as it may, shouldn't something be said about joining the Sirtfood diet with work out, is it fitting to stay away from practice totally or present it once you have begun the diet?

The SirtDiet Principles

With an expected 650 million hefty grown-ups internationally, it's critical to discover smart dieting and exercise systems that are feasible, don't deny you of all that you appreciate, and don't expect you to practice all week. The Sirtfood diet does only that. The thought is that sure nourishments will dynamic the 'thin quality' pathways which are normally actuated by fasting and exercise. Fortunately certain nourishment and drink, including dull chocolate and red wine, contain synthetic substances called polyphenols that enact the qualities that copy the impacts of activity and fasting.

Exercise during the initial barely any weeks

During the main week or two of the diet where your calorie admission is diminished, it is reasonable to stop or lessen practice while your body adjusts to less calories. Tune in to your body and if you feel exhausted or have less vitality than expected, don't work out. Rather guarantee that you stay concentrated on the rules that apply to a solid lifestyle, for example, including satisfactory day by day levels of fiber, protein and products of the soil.

When the diet turns into a lifestyle

When you do practice it's critical to devour protein in a perfect world an hour after your workout. Protein fixes muscles after exercise, lessens irritation and can help recuperation. There are an assortment of plans which incorporate protein which will be ideal for post-practice utilization, for example, the sirt stew con carne or the turmeric chicken and kale serving of mixed greens. If you need something lighter you could attempt the sirt blueberry smoothie and include some protein powder for included advantage. The kind of wellness you do will be down to you, however workouts at home will permit you to pick when to work out, the sorts of activities that suit you and are short and helpful.

The Sirtfood diet is incredible approach to change your dietary patterns, shed pounds and feel more advantageous. The underlying not many weeks may challenge you yet it's imperative to check which nourishments are ideal to eat and which scrumptious plans suit you. Be benevolent to yourself in the initial barely any weeks while your body adjusts and take practice simple if you decide to do it by any stretch of the imagination. If you are as of now somebody who moderates or extreme exercise then it might be that you can carry on as ordinary, or deal with your wellness as per the adjustment in diet. Similarly as with any diet and exercise changes, it's about the individual and how far you can propel yourself.

Minerals and nutrients for which ladies may require supplements incorporate calcium, iron, Vitamins B6, B12 and D. Men, be that as it may, need to focus on fiber, magnesium, Vitamins B9, C and E.

That reason applies to weight loss diets also. People's nourishment necessities sway which weight loss diets are increasingly compelling for each sex.

If you're similar to the vast majority, you've seen an astounding number of weight loss projects and patterns go back and forth; practically every one of them have their benefits and practically every one of them work — incidentally. Weight the executives and therapeutic experts fight collectively that the deep rooted, proven blend of good sustenance and ordinary exercise is the most ideal approach to adequately shed pounds and keep it off.

The Sirtfood Diet: For Women Only?

When the Sirtfood Diet started slanting, ladies all around hurled a murmur of delight. At last! Not just authorization to enjoy the two most pleasurable edibles on the planet — dull chocolate and red wine — yet support and justification! Then again, men may survey the diet and ask, "Where's the meat?"

"Sirtfood" is nourishment high in sirtuin proteins. The super-nourishments that are remembered for the Sirtfood Diet include:

- Apples
- Blueberries
- Buckwheat
- Capers
- Citrus natural products
- Dark chocolate in any event 85% cacao
- Extra-virgin olive oil
- Green tea
- Kale
- Medjool dates
- Parsley
- Red onions
- Red wine
- Rocket
- Turmeric
- Walnuts

It's accounted for that a diet high in these "super-nourishments" will:

- Burn fat
- Increase bulk
- Regulate digestion

The Diet — Phase 1

For three days, limit calories to 1,000/day and limit nourishments to three sirtfood green juices or smoothies (any blend of celery, kale, parsley) and 1 dinner/day sirfood-rich (turkey/chicken with escapades, parsley, sage). Starting on day 4 through day seven, increment calories to 1,500/day with 2 sirtfood green juices or smoothies and 2 sirtfood-rich dinners/day.

The Diet — Phase 2

For the accompanying two weeks, you'll consider a to be weight loss as you eat 3 sirtfood-rich dinners every day and one sirtfood green juice or smoothie.

How Is This Diet Different?

The Sirtfood Diet is different from different diets you've attempted in light of the fact that you won't see emotional weight loss. Defenders state you'll see strong weight loss that is consistent and offers the guarantee of long haul benefits. Similarly as with any dietary shift, you ought to counsel with your GP or restorative specialist before starting the Sirtfood Diet.

You'll discover plans in abundance on the web or can make your own utilizing lean meat, foods grown from the ground. Sides can remember seared red onion for olive oil, buckwheat and steamed kale.

At Holmes Place, we accept people's nourishment is critical to in general health. Our main goal is to urge and move individuals to diet, practice and create pressure decrease abilities, as per what is refreshing for every person. Make certain to investigate our site for extraordinary formula thoughts.

CONCLUSION

Stage one, before the diet really began, was to peruse The Sirtfood Diet and make a basic food item list. On the initial three days of the program I would gulp down three green juices — made up of kale, arugula, ginger, green apple, parsley, lemon and macha powder — and only one supper for every day. This ought to have set off a monster warning for me, yet the dinners I got sounded extraordinary — miso and sesame-coated tofu with ginger and bean stew sautéed greens, shrimp pan sear with buckwheat noodles — in addition to following three days you go up to two suppers every day, and two green juices. So I joyfully headed out to Whole Foods.

The plans fortunately are loaded up with fixings you can discover at any market, anyplace in the nation — aside from a certain something: buckwheat. I was unable to discover it on my first shopping excursion (the main motivation behind why I went to Whole Foods for my goods in any case), and it took me another two attempts to at long last find the grain (much obliged, Chelsea Whole Foods!).

Buckwheat and the different sirtfoods are the central purposes of the diet since they're high in polyphenols — a plant-based supplement that Goggins and Matten state are extraordinary for the stomach related framework.

Polyphenols "actuate an incredible reusing process in the body which gets out cell waste and consumes fat," the couple write in the book. "They do this by actuating our sirtuin qualities — otherwise called our 'thin' qualities. Undoubtedly, these are exactly the same qualities that are initiated by fasting and exercise."

Day 1:

That morning, superbly content subsequent to making the most of my typical three (solid ish!) suppers the day preceding, I aired out my first green juice to begin the diet (I will concede here that I conned a piece from the beginning — I don't have a juicer, nor the space in my loft to store one, so I purchased juices that coordinated the fixings in Sirtfood's formula from Juice Press and Pressed Juicery in New York City). Quite great! I've never been a customary green juice-consumer, however this was pleasant enough.

I continued tasting for the duration of the day, and began getting my typical craving calls around 11 a.m. I have a quite extreme nibble enslavement, yet I in any event go for the sound stuff, similar to pistachios and granola bars, and this was ordinarily when I get my fix. Be that as it may, I pushed through. Goggins and Matten state that you can eat your one feast whenever of the day, so I chose to go for 4 p.m.

By 1 p.m., I was hopeless and starving. The green juice did literally nothing to control my appetite, which bodes well — nothing in it has genuine backbone. I routinely compose the What I Eat segments, and I continued intuition about the nutritionists who talk about the requirement for dinners with protein to keep you fulfilled, something I was seriously deficient. My day accumulated, so I some way or another didn't really eat until 5 p.m. Fortunately, the supper was DELICIOUS. I went for the previously mentioned miso-coated tofu, and I would make this anytime. I even figured out how to spare piece of it to eat when I returned home from work as a "supper" (is it against the guidelines to separate the one feast? I was too ravenous to even think about caring).

The Sirtfood Diet

Day 2:

Increasingly green juice. More yearning.

The present feast was harissa-heated tofu with cauliflower "couscous." I'm not veggie lover, yet I'm not a major devotee of shrimp, the other alternative that day. I likely ought to have gone with it at any rate however — this supper was a major miss for me. It again needed anything fulfilling, so I was hopeless the whole day, especially when I gravely followed my companions to supper at Sweetgreen (most likely my untouched most loved quick easygoing eatery) that night and tasted the omnipresent green squeeze as they chomped on plates of mixed greens. Truly, I was desirous of servings of mixed greens.

Day 3:

You got it! I had green juice for breakfast.

My supper today was a kale and red onion dal with buckwheat, and WOW. I cherished it. I needed heaps of it. Be that as it may, my one bit was shockingly fulfilling — I think now my craving had gone down from eating under 1,000 calories every day, in addition to the dal included a lot of satisfying fixings, similar to lentils, buckwheat (I discovered it!) and solid fat-filled coconut milk. I don't gauge myself, however by day three I was easily wearing my most secure pair of thin pants, and my typically adjusted stomach was a lot compliment.

The main residual issue? I'm somebody who practices routinely, and hard. I go to CrossFit three times each week, once in a while more, and I run or swim on different days. With such a low carbohydrate content, that wasn't prescribed (I messaged Goggins, who stated, "The gentle calorie limitation in addition to the high admission of sirtuin-initiating supplements is making a mellow weight on our cells which causes sirtuin action to emphatically kick in. An excessive amount of activity worthwhile motivations an excessive amount of pressure, which could then be unfavorable"), however I love the head-freeing profits by work out. I went to CrossFit that night, and realizing I needed to go again in the first part of the day for the standard Saturday workout, I hard-bubbled two eggs and ate them with Old Bay and showered extra-virgin olive oil, my top pick. It was past important.

Day 4:

I could at last eat two dinners per day — yippee! In any case, my intense workout obviously turned out poorly on such little nourishment in the course of the most recent three days. So with the expansion in nourishment on the arrangement, I chose to change it up — I would return to eating regularly, and simply evaluate different plans for the remainder of the week. I'm difficult and profoundly serious, so it was disappointing to "come up short" at the diet, yet I likewise incredibly love nourishment, and skirting one to two dinners daily was not justified, despite any potential benefits to me.

The remainder of the week:

Different dinners I attempted — sautéed salmon with caramelized endive, arugula and celery leaf serving of mixed greens (it additionally has avocado!); Tuscan bean stew; the sirt super plate of mixed greens; the sirtfood omelet — were all comparatively phenomenal. I need to give a generous props to Goggins and Matten for making plans that are heavenly and loaded up with ordinary fixings — in addition to they were often one-container dinners, which is key for somebody without a dishwasher nor an individual to do the dishes for you (which I'm obviously expecting Adele has — livin' the fantasy).

The Verdict:

If you are insusceptible to hunger and truly appreciate green juices, put it all on the line (and check with your primary care physician beforehand)! If you're increasingly similar to me, skip week one, and go directly to week two, when you find a workable pace full and really fantastic dinners daily. Furthermore, you can in any case claim to be Adele.

SIRTFOOD DIET COOKBOOK

THE NUTRITION GUIDE FOR HEALTHY WEIGHT LOSS AND WELLBEING. EXCLUSIVE RECIPES AND MEAL PLAN TO ACTIVATE YOUR SKINNY GENE, BURN FAT AND EAT SMART EVERYDAY. LOSE 7 LBS IN 7 DAYS

Isabel Taylor

INTRODUCTION

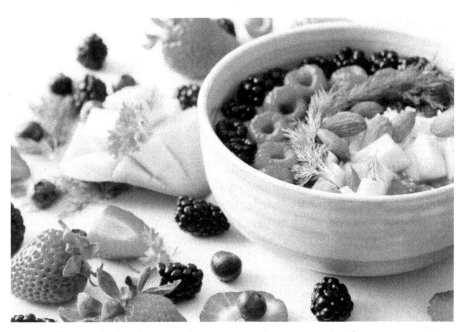

Regardless of whether you're attempting to get in shape or getting increasingly careful about energizing your body, it's essential to comprehend Sirtfoods. Sirtfoods are a gathering of nourishments wealthy in supplements that help manage your digestion, consume fat, and increment muscle. Aidan Goggins and Glen Matten, creators of THE SIRTFOOD DIET, share what you have to think about Sirtfoods.

When we cut back on calories, it makes a lack of vitality that enacts what is known as the "thin quality." This triggers a heap of positive changes. It places the body into a sort of endurance mode where it quits putting away fat and ordinary development forms are required to be postponed momentarily. Rather, the body directs its concentration toward consuming its stores of fat and turning on amazing housekeeping qualities that fix and restore our phones, successfully giving them a spring cleaning. The end result is weight loss and improved protection from ailment.

Be that as it may, the same number of dieters know, cutting calories includes some significant downfalls. Temporarily, the decrease in vitality consumption incites hunger, crabbiness, weakness, and muscle loss. Longer-term calorie limitation makes our digestion stagnate. This is the defeat of all calorie-prohibitive diets and makes ready for the weight to return heaping on. It is thus that 99 percent of dieters are destined to bomb over the long haul.

The entirety of this drove us to pose a major inquiry: is it by one way or another conceivable to actuate our thin quality with all the extraordinary advantages that brings without expecting to adhere to exceptional calorie limitation with every one of those downsides?

Enter Sirtfoods, a newfound gathering of marvel nourishments. Sirtfoods are especially wealthy in uncommon supplements that, when we expend them, can initiate a similar thin quality in our bodies that calorie limitation does. These qualities are known as sirtuins. They previously became known in a milestone study in 2003 when scientists found that resveratrol, a compound found in red grape skin and red wine, significantly expanded the life range of yeast.2 Incredibly, resveratrol had a similar impact on life span as calorie limitation, yet this was accomplished without lessening vitality admission. From that point forward investigations have indicated that resveratrol can expand

life in worms, flies, fish, and even honeybees.3 And from mice to people, beginning time examines show resveratrol secures against the unfriendly impacts of unhealthy, high-fat, and high-sugar diets; advances sound maturing by deferring age-related sicknesses; and increments fitness.4 basically it has been appeared to impersonate the impacts of calorie limitation and exercise.

With its rich resveratrol content, red wine was hailed as the first Sirtfood, clarifying the medical advantages connected to its utilization, and even why individuals who drink red wine increase less weight. However, this is just the start of the Sirtfood story.

With the revelation of resveratrol, the universe of wellbeing research was on the cusp of something significant, and the pharmaceutical business burned through no time committing. Scientists started screening a huge number of different synthetic substances for their capacity to initiate our sirtuin qualities. This uncovered various characteristic plant mixes, not only resveratrol, with significant sirtuin-actuating properties. It was additionally found that a given nourishment could contain an entire range of these plant mixes, which could work in show to both guide retention and amplify that nourishment's sirtuin-enacting impact. This had been one of the huge riddles around resveratrol. The researchers trying different things with resveratrol often expected to use far higher dosages than we know give an advantage when expended as a major aspect of red wine. In any case, just as resveratrol, red wine contains a variety of other regular plant mixes, including high measures of piceatannol just as quercetin, myricetin, and epicatechin, every one of which was appeared to autonomously initiate our sirtuin qualities and, progressively significant, to work in coordination.

The issue for the pharmaceutical business is that they can't advertise a gathering of supplements or nourishments as the following huge blockbuster sedate. So, all things being equal they contributed a huge number of dollars to create and direct preliminaries of manufactured mixes with expectations of revealing a Shangri-la pill. At this moment various investigations of sirtuin-enacting drugs are in progress for a huge number of interminable maladies, just as the first-since forever FDA-endorsed preliminary to examine whether a prescription can slow maturing.

As tempting as that may appear, if history has shown us anything, it's that we ought not hold out a lot of trust in this pharmaceutical ambrosia. Consistently the pharmaceutical and wellbeing enterprises have attempted to copy the advantages of nourishments and diets through segregated medications and supplements. What's more, on numerous occasions it's missed the mark. Why sit tight ten or more years for the permitting of these supposed marvel drugs, and the unavoidable reactions they bring, when right now we have all the staggering advantages accessible readily available through the nourishment we eat?

So, while the pharmaceutical business perseveringly seeks after a druglike enchantment slug, we need to retrain our emphasis on diet.

WHAT ARE SIRTFOOD?

While the world has been hanging tight for Adele to drop new music, it's been getting only somewhat fixated on her weight. There's no uncertainty that she looks extraordinary (um, hasn't she generally?) and it's reputed to be down to the Sirtfood Diet.

Lexi Larson, a 19-year-old from Hingham, Massachusetts, revealed to People that she met Adele on an extended get-away in Anguilla and that the music whiz disclosed to her she had "lost something like 100 pounds," portraying it as an "insane constructive encounter."

Adele hasn't affirmed that her weight loss is down to the Sirtfood Diet (or some other diet), however she is highlighted on the authority Sirtfood Diet site with the words, "Adele's top-mystery fat-softening diet."

So, what's the serious deal about the Sirtfood Diet?

The eating plan depends on polyphenols, characteristic mixes found in plant nourishments that help to shield the cells in the body from aggravation or demise through sickness. According to wellbeing advisors Aidan Goggins and Glen Matten, who formulated the Sirtfood Diet, a little gathering of polyphenols can imitate the impacts of fasting and exercise by initiating the body's sirtuin (otherwise known as "thin") qualities.

"In view of expending a specific rundown of solid, polyphenol-rich nourishments, the Sirtfood Diet guarantees weight and fat decrease without muscle loss," says New York-based dietitian-nutritionist Tanya Freirich, RD, at Sweet Nova.

What's the arrangement?

There are two stages to the Sirtfood diet; the primary goes on for multi week and the second for about fourteen days. During the initial three days of the arrangement, you're confined to 1,000 calories from one feast of sirtfoods and three green juices. For the remainder of the primary week, you can devour two green juices and two sirtfood dinners for every day. During stage two, the day by day feast plan comprises of three sirtfood dinners and one green juice.

Adjusted sirtfood-rich dinners incorporate Asian Shrimp Stir-Fry with Buckwheat Noodles and Strawberry Buckwheat Tabbouleh.

Past the underlying three-week "kick off" period, Goggins and Matten prescribe proceeding to incorporate sirtfoods in your dinners to keep getting results.

What does it guarantee?

"If you don't veer off from the arrangement, the Sirtfood Diet guarantees a seven-pound weight loss in the primary week (without losing bulk)," says Freirich. "It additionally claims to have hostile to maturing impacts, to help improve memory and glucose control and lessen the danger of ceaseless ailment."

In any case, does it convey?

The examination on the job of sirtuin is really meager—for the most part research center investigations including yeast, lab creatures, and human undeveloped cells. One examination, distributed in 2013 in the diary Oxidative Medicine and Cellular Longevity, proposes polyphenol utilization has a similar advantageous impact on human digestion as calorie limitation. However, until this dietary methodology is really tried in human clinical preliminaries, it's difficult to state with any assurance how individuals may toll.

What would you be able to eat?

While some sirtfoods are standard in any grocery store or wellbeing nourishment store (and may as of now be in your kitchen), others may not be so natural to discover.

"Sirtfoods incorporate kale, dull chocolate, red wine, cocoa powder, turmeric, onions, parsley, garlic, pecans, and strawberries," Freirich says. "A large portion of the fixings are anything but difficult to discover and are notable as solid decisions. In any case, extra fixings might be more enthusiastically to source, similar to lovage, buckwheat, and matcha green tea powder."

What wouldn't you be able to eat?

Formally, no nourishments are "prohibited" on the Sirtfood Diet, yet the calorie limitation is not kidding—especially during the underlying three days, when you're constrained to 1,000 calories.

To place that in context, 1,000 calories is the prescribed admission for an inactive 2-to 3-year-old, according to the USDA Dietary Guidelines for 2015-2020,

Are there any disadvantages?

The hardest piece of the Sirtfood Diet is calorie limitation and the dependence on green juice, and this could be perilous for specific gatherings of individuals, Freirich says. She wouldn't prescribe this diet for individuals on certain drugs, similar to Coumadin, or with wellbeing conditions like diabetes. She'd likewise give it a miss if you're preparing broadly or are pregnant or breastfeeding.

"By and large, I don't suggest any diets that depend on excessively prohibitive outside principles," Freirich includes. "Be that as it may, a significant number of the suggested 'sirtfoods' are wellbeing advancing, and I'd prescribe individuals consolidate these in their dinners. As usual, I emphatically urge individuals to tune in to their body's craving and satiety signals for direction on when and how much nourishment to eat."

LOSE SEVEN POUNDS IN SEVEN DAYS WITH THE SOLID ROUTE ON THE SIRTFOOD DIET RECIPE

According to an ongoing review, the normal lady increases 5lb in pre-winter, while December is the fattest month of the year.

Ut if every one of those pumpkin flavor lattes in the course of the most recent couple of months mean you're breaking a rib attempting to press into your LBD in time for the workplace party, the current year's most discussed diet guarantees that you can shed 7lb in only seven days, keep the weight off and still have chocolate.

It might sound unrealistic, however superstars, for example, Adele, Lorraine Pascale and Jodie Kidd depend on the Sirtfood Diet.

"A sirtfood is high in sirtuin activators," clarifies nutritionist Aidan Goggins, co-writer of the top of the line book The Sirtfood Diet.

"Sirtuins are a kind of protein that shield cells from kicking the bucket or getting aggravated. They can likewise launch your digestion, control your hunger, help muscle tone and consume fat."

So, how can it work?

"For the initial three days, you confine calorie admission to 1,000 calories every day, which incorporates drinking three sirtfood green juices in addition to eating

a sirtfood-rich feast and nibbling on cell reinforcement stuffed 'sirtfood chomps'," says Aidan.

"Throughout the previous four days, you up the calorie admission to 1,500 calories per day by expending two sirtfood-rich dinners and two green juices, removing the chomps."

What's to come

You can do this arrangement for as long as about fourteen days, after which it's tied in with modifying it to suit your lifestyle.

"There are no set guidelines – simply attempt to incorporate however many sirtfoods as could be allowed in your diet, which should cause you to feel more beneficial, increasingly vivacious and improve your skin, just as making you slenderer," says Aidan.

"Customers who have continued with the diet have seen proceeded and supported weight loss of over 2st."

Your seven-day plan

This super-sound green juice and these yummy choc balls are Sirtfood Diet staples.

All plans serve one (except if in any case expressed).

Sirtfood Green Juice

*75g kale

*30g rocket

*5g level leaf parsley

*5g lovage leaves (discretionary)

*150g celery, including leaves

*1/2 medium green apple

*Juice 1/2 lemon

*1/2tsp matcha green tea

1 Juice the kale, rocket, parsley and lovage, if utilizing, then include the celery and apple and mix once more. Press in the lemon.

2 Pour a modest quantity of the juice into a glass, then include the matcha and mix until broke up. Include the rest of the juice and serve right away.

NOTE Only use matcha in the initial two beverages of the day, as it contains a similar caffeine content as a typical cup of tea. If you're not accustomed to it, it might keep you conscious if alcoholic later in the day.

Sirtfood Bites (makes 15-20 chomps)

*120g pecans

*30g dull chocolate (85% cocoa solids), broken into pieces, or cocoa nibs

*250g Medjool dates, pitted

*1tbsp cocoa powder

*1tbsp ground turmeric

*1tbsp additional virgin olive oil

*Scraped seeds of 1 vanilla unit or 1tsp vanilla concentrate

1 Place the pecans and chocolate into a nourishment processor and mix until you have a fine powder. Include the various fixings and mix until the blend shapes an enormous ball. Add 2tbsp water to help tie it, if required.

2 Using your hands, make scaled down balls from the blend and refrigerate in an impermeable holder for at any rate 1 hour before serving. The balls will keep for as long as seven days in the ice chest.

Day 1

3 x sirtfood green juices

2 x sirtfood chomps (you can substitute these for 15-20g of dull chocolate if you wish)

1 x sirtfood supper

Asian lord prawn pan sear

*150g crude ruler prawns, shelled

*2tsp tamari or soy sauce

*2tsp additional virgin olive oil

*1 clove garlic, finely hacked

*1 10,000 foot stew, finely slashed

*1tsp new ginger, finely hacked

*20g red onion, cut

*40g celery, cut and cut

*75g green beans, hacked

*50g kale, generally hacked

*100ml chicken stock

*75g soba (buckwheat noodles)

*5g lovage or celery leaves

1 In a skillet over a high warmth, cook the prawns in 1tsp tamari or soy sauce and 1tsp oil for 2-3 minutes. Move to a plate.

2 Add the rest of the oil to the dish and fry the garlic, stew, ginger, red onion, celery, beans and kale over a medium-high warmth for 2-3 minutes. Add the stock and bring to the bubble, then stew until the vegetables are cooked yet at the same time crunchy.

3 Cook the noodles in bubbling water according to pack directions. Channel and include the lovage or celery leaves, noodles and prawns to the container. Take back to the bubble, then expel from the warmth and serve.

Day 2

*3 x sirtfood green juices

*2 x sirtfood nibbles

*1 x sirtfood feast

Turkey escalope

*150g cauliflower, generally slashed

*1 clove garlic, finely slashed

*40g red onion, finely slashed

*1 superior stew, finely hacked

*1tsp crisp ginger, finely hacked

*2tbsp additional virgin olive oil

*2tsp ground turmeric

*30g sun-dried tomatoes, finely hacked

*10g parsley

*150g turkey escalope

*1tsp dried sage

*Juice 1/2 lemon

*1tbsp tricks

1 Place the cauliflower in a nourishment processor and heartbeat in 2-second blasts to finely cleave it until it looks like couscous. Put in a safe spot. Fry the garlic, red onion, bean stew and ginger in 1tsp of the oil until delicate however not hued. Include the turmeric and cauliflower and cook for 1 moment. Expel from the warmth and include the sun-dried tomatoes and a large portion of the parsley.

2 Coat the turkey escalope in the rest of the oil and sage then fry for 5-6 minutes, turning normally. When cooked, include the lemon juice, remaining parsley, tricks and 1tbsp water to the container to make a sauce, then serve.

Day 3

3 x sirtfood green juices

2 x sirtfood chomps

1 x sirtfood dinner

Fragrant chicken

For the salsa

*1 huge tomato

*1 10,000 foot bean stew, finely cleaved

*1tbsp tricks, finely cleaved

*5g parsley, finely hacked

*Juice 1/2 lemon

For the chicken

*120g skinless, boneless chicken bosom

*2tsp ground turmeric

*Juice 1/2 lemon

*1tbsp additional virgin olive oil

*50g kale, hacked

*20g red onion, cut

*1tsp new ginger, finely cleaved

*50g buckwheat

1 Heat the stove to 220°C/200°C fan/gas mark 7.

2 To make the salsa, finely slash the tomato, ensuring you keep however much of the fluid as could reasonably be expected. Blend in with the bean stew, tricks, parsley and lemon juice.

3 Marinate the chicken bosom in 1tsp of the turmeric, lemon juice and a large portion of the oil for 5-10 minutes.

4 Heat an ovenproof griddle, include the marinated chicken and cook for a moment on each side until brilliant, then exchange to the broiler for 8-10 minutes or until cooked through. Expel, spread with foil and leave to rest for 5 minutes.

5 Cook the kale in a steamer for 5 minutes. Fry the onion and ginger in the remainder of the oil until delicate yet not shaded, then include the cooked kale and fry for one more moment.

6 Cook the buckwheat according to pack directions with the rest of the turmeric and serve.

Day 4

2 x sirtfood green juices

2 x sirtfood dinners

Sirt Muesli

*20g buckwheat chips

*10g buckwheat puffs

*15g coconut chips or dried up coconut

*40g Medjool dates, hollowed and hacked

*15g pecans, hacked

*10g cocoa nibs

*100g strawberries, hulled and hacked

*100g plain Greek yogurt (or veggie lover elective, for example, soya or coconut yogurt)

1 Mix the entirety of the fixings together and serve (forgetting about the strawberries and yogurt if not serving straight away).

Sautéed salmon serving of mixed greens

For the dressing

*10g parsley

*Juice 1/2 lemon

*1tbsp tricks

*1tbsp additional virgin olive oil

For the serving of mixed greens

*1/2 avocado, stripped, stoned and diced

*100g cherry tomatoes, divided

*20g red onion, meagerly cut

*50g rocket

*5g celery leaves

*150g skinless salmon filet

*2tsp darker sugar

*70g chicory (head), divided lengthways

1 Heat the broiler to 220ºC/200ºC fan/gas mark 7.

2 To make the dressing, whizz the parsley, lemon juice, tricks and 2tsp oil in a blender until smooth.

3 For the plate of mixed greens, blend the avocado, tomato, red onion, rocket and celery leaves together.

4 Rub the salmon with a little oil and singe it in an ovenproof skillet for a moment. Move to a heating plate and cook in the broiler for 5 minutes.

5 Mix the darker sugar with 1tsp oil and brush it over the cut sides of the chicory. Spot chop sides down in a hot skillet and cook for 2-3 minutes, turning normally. Dress the plate of mixed greens and serve together.

Day 5

2 x sirtfood green juices

2 x sirtfood dinners

Strawberry tabbouleh

*50g buckwheat

*1tbsp ground turmeric

*80g avocado

*65g tomato

*20g red onion

*25g Medjool dates, pitted

*1tbsp tricks

*30g parsley

*100g strawberries, hulled

*1tbsp additional virgin olive oil

*Juice 1/2 lemon

*30g rocket

1 Cook the buckwheat with the turmeric according to pack guidelines. Channel and cool.

2 Finely cleave the avocado, tomato, red onion, dates, tricks and parsley and blend in with the cooled buckwheat.

3 Slice the strawberries and delicately blend into the plate of mixed greens with the oil and lemon juice. Serve on the rocket.

Miso-marinated prepared cod

*20g miso

*1tbsp mirin

*1tbsp additional virgin olive oil

*200g skinless cod filet

*20g red onion, cut

*40g celery, cut

*1 clove garlic, finely hacked

*1 10,000 foot bean stew, finely cleaved

*1tsp new ginger, finely slashed

*60g green beans

*50g kale, generally hacked

*30g buckwheat

*1tsp ground turmeric

*1tsp sesame seeds

*5g parsley, generally hacked

*1tbsp tamari or soy sauce

1 Heat the stove to 220°C/200°C fan/gas mark 7.

2 Mix the miso, mirin and 1tsp oil, rub into the cod and marinate for 30 minutes. Move on to a heating plate and cook for 10 minutes.

3 Meanwhile, heat an enormous skillet with the rest of the oil. Include the onion and sautéed food for a couple of moments, then include the celery, garlic, stew, ginger, green beans and kale. Fry until the kale is delicate and cooked through, adding a little water to soften the kale if required.

4 Cook the buckwheat according to pack directions with the turmeric. Include the sesame seeds, parsley and tamari or soy sauce to the pan fried food and present with the greens and fish.

Day 6

2 x sirtfood green juices

2 x sirtfood dinners

Sirt super plate of mixed greens

*50g rocket

*50g chicory leaves

*100g smoked salmon cuts

*80g avocado, stripped, stoned and cut

*40g celery, cut

*20g red onion, cut

*15g pecans, hacked

*1tbsp tricks

*1 huge Medjool date, hollowed and slashed

*1tbsp additional virgin olive oil

*Juice 1/2 lemon

*10g parsley, cleaved

*10g lovage or celery leaves, cleaved

1 Mix every one of the fixings together and serve.

Chargrilled meat

*100g potatoes, stripped and diced into 2cm 3D shapes

*1tbsp additional virgin olive oil

*5g parsley, finely cleaved

*50g red onion, cut into rings

*50g kale, cleaved

*1 clove garlic, finely cleaved

*120-150g 3.5cm-thick meat filet steak or 2cm-thick sirloin steak

*40ml red wine

*150ml meat stock

*1tsp tomato purée

*1tsp cornflour, broke down in 1tbsp water

1 Heat the stove to 220°C/200°C fan/gas mark 7.

2 Place the potatoes in a pan of bubbling water, bring to the bubble and cook for 4-5 minutes, then channel. Spot in a simmering tin with 1tsp oil and cook for 35-45 minutes, turning at regular intervals. Expel from the stove, sprinkle with the cleaved parsley and blend well.

3 Fry the onion in 1tsp oil over a medium warmth until delicate and caramelized. Keep warm.

4 Steam the kale for 2-3 minutes, then channel. Fry the garlic delicately in 1/2tsp oil for 1 moment until delicate. Include the kale and fry for a further 1-2 minutes, until delicate. Keep warm.

5 Heat an ovenproof griddle until smoking. Coat the meat in 1/2tsp oil and fry according to how you like your meat done. Expel from the dish and put aside to rest. Add the wine to the hot skillet to raise any meat buildup. Air pocket to decrease the wine considerably until it's syrupy with a concentrated flavor.

6 Add the stock and tomato purée to the steak container and bring to the bubble, then add the cornflour glue to thicken the sauce a little at once until you have the ideal consistency. Mix in any juice from the refreshed steak and present with the potatoes, kale, onion rings and red wine sauce.

Day 7

2 x sirtfood green juices

2 x sirtfood dinners

Sirtfood omelet

*50g streaky bacon

*3 medium eggs

*35g red chicory, daintily cut

*5g parsley, finely cleaved

*1tsp additional virgin olive oil

1 Heat a non-stick skillet. Cut the bacon into slight strips and cook over a high warmth until fresh. You don't have to include any oil – there ought to be sufficient fat in the bacon to cook it. Expel from the dish and spot on kitchen paper to deplete any abundance fat. Wipe the container clean.

2 Whisk the eggs and blend in with the chicory and parsley. Mix the cooked bacon through the eggs.

3 Heat the oil in a non-stick griddle before including the egg blend. Cook until the omelet solidifies. Facilitate the spatula around the edges and overlay the omelet down the middle or move up and serve.

Prepared chicken bosom

For the pesto

*15g parsley

*15g pecans

*15g Parmesan

*1tbsp additional virgin olive oil

*Juice 1/2 lemon

For the chicken

*150g skinless chicken bosom

*20g red onions, finely cut

*1tsp red wine vinegar

*35g rocket

*100g cherry tomatoes, split

*1tsp balsamic vinegar

1 Heat the stove to 220°C/200°C fan/gas mark 7.

2 To make the pesto, mix the parsley, pecans, Parmesan, olive oil, a large portion of the lemon juice and 1tbsp water in a nourishment processor until you have

a smooth glue. Step by step include more water until you have your favored consistency.

3 Marinate the chicken bosom in 1tbsp of the pesto and the rest of the lemon squeeze in the cooler for 30 minutes, or more if conceivable.

4 In an ovenproof griddle over a medium-high warmth, fry the chicken in its marinade for 1 moment on either side, then exchange the skillet to the stove and cook for 8 minutes, or until cooked through.

5 Marinate the onions in the red wine vinegar for 5-10 minutes, then channel off the fluid.

6 When the chicken is cooked, expel it from the stove, spoon over 1tbsp pesto and let the warmth from the chicken dissolve the pesto. Spread with foil and leave to rest for 5 minutes before serving.

7 Combine the rocket, tomatoes and onion and shower over the balsamic. Present with the chicken, spooning throughout the remainder of the pesto.

Need to continue onward? Throughout the following 14 days, have 1 x green juice and 3 x sirtfood-rich dinners daily.

Sirtfood Diet for Weight Loss: Lose 3 Kgs In A Week with This Diet Which Allows Red Wine and Chocolate! Sirtfood diet for weight loss: Turmeric, onion, dim chocolate, red wine, dates, pecans and buckwheat are a portion of the nourishments you can eat right now. Peruse here to know how it can assist you with weight loss

It depends on eating a gathering of nourishments that contain something the creators portray as 'sirtuin activators'. Sirtuins are a class of protein, seven of which (SIRT1 to SIRT7) have been identified in people. They seem to have a wide scope of jobs in our body, including potential enemy of maturing and metabolic impacts.

As researchers see progressively about sirtuins, they're getting inspired by the job they may play in assisting with turning on those weight-loss pathways that are generally activated by an absence of nourishment and by taking activity. The hypothesis goes that if you can initiate a portion of the seven sirtuins, you could assist with consuming fat and treat corpulence with less exertion than it takes to follow some different diets or go through hours on the treadmill.

What does it include?

The Sirtfood Diet has two phases. On every one of the initial three days you drink three 'sirt juices' and have one feast (aggregate of 1,000 calories per day). On the accompanying four days you're permitted two sirt juices and two suppers every day (aggregate of 1,500 calories day by day). You then advancement to the simpler stage two, with one juice and three 'adjusted' suppers, in reasonable segment measures, a day.

What would you be able to eat on the diet?

There's a rundown of nourishments containing synthetic exacerbates that the creators state switch on sirtuin and wrench up fat consuming while at the same time bringing down hunger (the last presumably through assisting with accomplishing better glucose control).

Nourishments include: strawberries, pecans, parsley, kale, rocket, espresso, green tea, turmeric, soy, escapades, 10,000 foot chillies, red onion, extra-virgin olive oil, celery, medjool dates, buckwheat, red wine – and, the most well-known sirtfood on the square, cocoa (deciphered, obviously, into dull chocolate). Sirt juices are produced using kale, celery, apple, lemon, matcha green tea, rocket and parsley. Run of the mill fundamental dinners incorporate Asian lord prawn pan sear with buckwheat noodles, and kale and red onion dahl with buckwheat.

Is it powerful for weight loss?

You ought to get in shape basically on the grounds that you're eating less calories, particularly in stage one. Without a doubt, you may consume fat quicker with this diet than with 'any old calorie-limited' plan and you may feel fuller. With respect to the creators' case this diet is 'clinically demonstrated to lose 7lb in seven days'...

All things considered, it's significant that so far the diet has just been tried on 40 solid, exceptionally energetic human guinea pigs in an upmarket rec center in London's Knightsbridge. The analyzers lost a normal of 7lb in seven days, while indicating increments in bulk and vitality. In any case, then given the calorie limitations of that first week, weight loss may basically be because of the outrageous decrease in calories.

The decision

Further examinations are expected to identify the long haul sway on waistlines – and general wellbeing – and to see whether sirt dieters keep the pounds off any more successfully than they would on different diets. We don't yet have the foggiest idea what, if any, sway the expansion of sirtfoods to our diet really has on our weight.

Furthermore, will anybody have the option to stay with the dreariness of juices and limit themselves to nourishments on the rundown (and be glad to dump their ordinary cuppa for green tea) for all time? With respect to the features that propose you can appreciate dull chocolate and red wine on this diet – well, truly, it is anything but a green light to devour heaps of either!

Cutting calories will consistently give you results

If you have the funds, the tendency and the stomach for it, I'm very certain it will 'work' somewhat for the time being, if simply because it's a compelling method to limit calories. Also, wine and chocolate aside, the rundown for the most part comprises of the very nourishments dietitians and nutritionists suggest for good wellbeing (think products of the soil!).

Regardless of whether it works all around ok to make it stand separated from a great many weight-loss designs that have trodden this tired way before likewise is not yet clear. It's reasonable Goggins and Matten will become smash hit diet creators, yet I think the uber bucks will truly stream once the pharmaceutical business figures out how to make sirtuin modulators that we can pop, so there'll be no compelling reason to down one more kale smoothie.

HOW DO SIRTFOOD AND DIET WORKS?

The Sirtfood Diet is developing in ubiquity, however does it truly work for weight loss? Sirtuins are characterized as a bunch of proteins that assume a fundamental job in cell wellbeing and direct different body capacities. These sirtuins may likewise assume a significant job in directing the digestion, fat consuming, expanding bulk and decreasing aggravation. According to sirtfood diet lovers, certain entire nourishments contain sirtfood activators that expansion these proteins in the body. A short rundown of well-known sirtfoods incorporates:

- Olive oil
- Turmeric
- Citrus organic products
- Kale
- Onions
- Buckwheat
- Matcha green tea
- Parsley
- Soy
- Pecans
- Arugula
- Green juice

One significant explanation the sirtfood diet has detonated in ubiquity is because of its stipend of dull chocolate and red wine, as the two things are considered sirtfoods. The case is that by concentrating on these nourishments, fast weight loss will follow without diminishes in bulk. A sirtfood dieter will start their first week drinking green juice made of matcha green tea, lemon juice, parsley, celery, a green apple and arugula three times each week. After the main week, sirtfood dieters come back to eating three suppers for each day made uniquely with sirtfoods and will keep on joining these nourishments all through the rest of the diet.

Does the Sirtfood Diet Actually Work?

There is by all accounts a developing number of famous people and remarkable figures who've touted the sirtfood diet for their ongoing weight loss achievement. Be that as it may, buyers must remember that famous people often approach proficient help when it comes to what they devour and any extra exercise regimens. Also, considers on the adequacy of this diet are thin. Without a doubt, most nourishments recorded are solid entire nourishment alternatives and calorie limitations which are consequently associated with some weight loss. Most of nourishments recorded have mitigating properties, high measures of cancer prevention agents and supplements which are obviously, helpful. Therapeutic specialists caution however, that while snappy weight loss is conceivable on such a diet, a larger part of that underlying loss will be water weight. It might likewise be hazardous for the individuals who take part in moderate to high physical movement.

While regimens like the sirtfood diet still can't seem to be demonstrated when it comes to feasible weight loss, restorative weight loss is a demonstrated and successful answer for any individual who has battled with weight changes and cycles. Diet Demand's primary care physician planned diets are altered to every person for protected, quickened results that lead to long haul achievement.

The most recent diet furor that is slanting among superstars is the sirtfood diet. The diet was brought to the spotlight by two VIP nutritionists in the UK who asserted it as a progressive new diet that works by turning on your "thin quality." according to their case, sirtfood diet can advance quick weight loss, while keeping up bulk and keep you from constant sickness.

How the Diet Works?

These uncommon nourishments initiate sirtuins (SIRTs), a gathering of seven proteins found in the body that manage digestion, irritation and the maturing procedure. These specific proteins are known to shield cells from passing on because of stress. Analysts accept sirtuins additionally improve the body's capacity to consume fat and lift digestion.

Certain plant mixes can build the degree of these proteins in the body. Nourishments containing these mixes are known as "sirtfoods." The Sirtfood diet plan is based around 20 food sources which incorporate kale, red wine, strawberries, onions, soy, parsley, additional virgin olive oil, dull chocolate (85% cocoa), matcha green tea, buckwheat, turmeric, pecans, arugula (rocket), elevated stew, lovage, medjool dates, red chicory, blueberries, escapades, espresso.

Need to Follow the Diet? Here Is How to Do It

The diet is the blend of sirtfoods and calorie limitation to build the degrees of sirtuins in the body. The diet book incorporates feast plans and plans to follow.

It is to be followed in two stages: The underlying stage which goes on for multi week includes limiting calories to 1000kcal for three days. During nowadays you need to drink three sirtfood green juices and one dinner daily that is rich in sirtfoods. During the remainder of the days (four to seven), calorie admission ought to be expanded to 1500kcal. This time you need to expend two sirtfood green juices and two sirtfood-rich dinners daily.

The subsequent stage, otherwise called the support stage, keeps going 14 days. This is where you can see relentless weight loss. During this period, you can eat three adjusted sirtfood-rich dinners consistently, in addition to one green juice. Much after the finish of these stages, the makers of the diet suggest proceeding sirtfoods and green juice into your standard diet.

Alert: There isn't a lot of verification to back this new diet pattern.

There are various craze diets out there. Everyone professes to be preferable and progressively viable over the other. If you are attempting to settle on the best diet plan that you can follow, we wager you are befuddled as hellfire. One diet that makes certain to confound you more than some other diet is most likely the Super Carb Diet. Carbs are given a wide compartment by practically all weight watchers. So how might we have a diet on carbs?

The Super Carb Diet was created by Bob Harper, a VIP mentor and host of The Biggest Loser. This diet looks to adjust the admission of proteins and fiber. It does as such by remembering complex starches and negligible fats for the diet. It can assist you with getting in shape adequately without causing you to feel denied.

Super Carb Foods

Nourishments like sweet potatoes, entire grains, lentils, beans, quinoa and couscous contain complex sound carbs. Dissimilar to refined carbs, there complex carbs hold glucose levels under control and actuates weight loss. You can likewise incorporate dark colored rice and cereal to your diet. Butternut squash, beets, cucumber and broccoli are pressed with sound carbs as are natural products like apples, grapes and bananas.

The Super Carb Diet Plan

Right now, need to keep away from entire grains and pasta during lunch and supper. You may have snacks between dinners, yet this can be just organic products or vegetables. To make the diet progressively successful, incorporate ginger, turmeric, garlic and cayenne to your diet. It will invigorate your digestion and lift absorption. Follow this diet for a month and see the difference.

Breakfast: You may have super grains like cereal, quinoa, an English biscuit or an entire grain tortilla for breakfast. Be that as it may, ensure you don't expend in excess of 300 calories.

Lunch and supper: Include boring vegetables and organic products like sweet potatoes, squash, broccoli, apples and grapes to your dinners. Additionally, include a segment of protein-rich nourishments like fish and eggs. Vegetarians can add tofu and yogurt to their diet. Ensure you limit your calorie admission to 400 and 500 calories each for lunch and supper individually.

It sounds unrealistic...

If someone educated, you concerning a diet that permits you to drink red wine and eat dull chocolate—while likewise shedding kilos like insane—your first inquiry may be: what's the trick?

Yet, evidently there isn't one, according to the makers of the Sirtfood Diet, the most recent weight-loss plan creating a ruckus on the interwebs and getting love on Instagram. That is on the grounds that wine and chocolate, alongside nourishments like strawberries, rocket pecans, and kale, are among an assortment of "Sirtfoods" that supposedly initiate your body's characteristic "thin qualities" to assist you with consuming fat.

It's unmistakable why this diet is so well known (see: wine, chocolate), however is it unrealistic? Here's all that you have to know.

What It Is

The creators of The Sirtfood Diet exhort eating nourishments rich in sirtuins, a sort of plant-based protein that has given some guarantee in clinical investigations to improve metabolic wellbeing. "The eating plan itself is intended to 'turn on' the sirtuin qualities (especially SIRT-1), which are accepted to support digestion, increment fat consuming, battle aggravation, and check hunger," says enrolled dietician, Edwina Clark, head of nourishment and health for Yummly.

Early examinations propose that kilojoule limitation and resveratrol (a polyphenol found in nourishments like grapes, blueberries, and peanuts), actuate the SIRT-1 quality, and these two standards support the Sirtfood way to deal with eating.

The diet endures a sum of three weeks and is isolated into two stages. During stage one, you restrict yourself to three Sirtfood green juices (containing kale, arugula, parsley, celery, green apple, lemon squeeze, and green tea) and one Sirtfood-rich supper every day, totalling around 4000 kilojoules every day, says Dr Caroline Apovian, chief of the Nutrition and Weight Management Center at the Boston Medical Center.

For the following four days, you drink two Sirtfood green squeezes and eat two Sirtfood-rich dinners, which brings your kilojoule aggregate to around 6000 every day.

Stage two, or the upkeep arrange, endures 14 days. During those two weeks, you should have three Sirtfood-rich suppers and one Sirtfood green squeeze day by day.

When those three weeks are up, there's no set intend to follow. To proceed on the Sirtfood way, you should simply change every one of your suppers to incorporate however many Sirtfoods as could be expected under the circumstances. Exercise is additionally supported (30 minutes of movement, five days per week), however getting sweat-soaked isn't the principle focal point of the weight-loss plan.

See probably the craziest diets individuals have really attempted:

Advantages and disadvantages

The Sirtfood Diet incorporates numerous nutritious nourishments that are advantageous for weight loss, for example, celery, kale, green tea, Medjool dates, lean chicken, lean red meat, and parsley, says Apovian. The diet additionally confines or kills numerous nourishments that are known to cause weight increase, for example, refined flours, included sugars, and handled nourishments with practically zero dietary benefit. What's more, because of that absurdly low kilojoule consumption, adherents will probably get in shape gave they stay on track, she says.

"Proof to date proposes that kilojoule limitation and irregular fasting can be a compelling procedure for weight loss and improving metabolic wellbeing," says Clark. "In any case, this may not be fitting for everybody," she says.

The long haul supportability of this arrangement is flawed. When you're past the initial not many weeks, there's no eating procedure to follow other than adding more Sirtfoods to every dinner. This makes the diet substantially more adaptable than most, which is a tremendous advantage, however a three-week extended length of hardship could without much of a stretch lead to indulging during stage two, eventually putting you back at the starting point.

As diets go, one that touts the advantages of red wine and dim chocolate utilization seems like a thick cut of dieting paradise. In any case, that is not everything to the most current U.K. big name diet pattern, the Sirtfood Diet.

The diet was created by creators and sustenance specialists Aidan Goggins and Glen Matten, who both learned at the University of Surrey and hold graduate degrees in healthful drug. In Goggins and Matten's book The Sirtfood Diet, they depict an eating plan that vows to "switch on your 'thin quality,'" or rather a class of qualities that code for sirtuins (SIRTs), which are proteins that help manage fat creation and capacity.

"We became charmed by the potential for specific nourishments to turn on a ground-breaking reusing process in the body that gets out cell waste and consumes fat. They do this by actuating the equivalent 'thin' qualities that are enacted by fasting and exercise. We call these nourishments sirtfoods," Matten says. "When we put these nourishments into an extraordinary Sirtfood Diet and trialed it, members shed seven pounds in seven days and detailed inclination the best they at any point had."

The book was distributed in January 2016 in the U.K. furthermore, Matten hopes to report the U.S. discharge "unavoidably."

The Science of the Sirtfood Diet (brief)

Expending nourishments rich in "sirtuin activators" — including red wine, kale, arugula, buckwheat, apples, blueberries, tricks, red onions, pecans, strawberries, additional virgin olive oil, parsley, dull chocolate, green tea, and espresso among others — should upregulate the outflow of SIRT qualities, expanding the creating sirtuin proteins that will (ideally) hinder the gathering of fat. You've likely known about the most celebrated of the sirtuin activators: Resveratrol, a compound found in red wine.

In 2003, David A. Sinclair, Ph.D., an educator in the Department of Genetics at Harvard Medical School, distributed the consequences of the principal concentrate to propose that resveratrol eases back maturing in a manner like calorie limitation — that is, by animating the SIRT2 quality, which advances DNA soundness, builds the generation of the body's own cancer prevention agents, and slows down fat creation. From that point forward, a lot more sirtuin activators (and the nourishments where they're found) have been identified, and the rundown of potential advantages from expending them continues developing.

Potential Benefits of the Sirtfood Diet

Sirtuins have additionally been attached to the working of the anxious, cardiovascular, and safe frameworks, just as liver, bone, muscle, foundational microorganism, and tissue recovery, according to 2014 article "The Controversial World of Sirtuins" distributed in the diary Drug Discovery Today: Technologies. Sirtuins have additionally been attributed with assisting with battling many age-related illnesses, including malignancy, cardiovascular sickness, metabolic issue, osteoporosis, neurodegenerative ailments, and joint inflammation.

Studies have additionally uncovered that sirtuins can diminish aggravation, hypoxic worry (as may be brought about by poor flow), heat stun, and genotoxic (DNA harming) worry, according to 2011 article "Sirtuins at a Glance" in the Journal of Cell Science, which takes note of that irritation is a significant reason for maturing and maturing related maladies.

Sirtfood Diet at a Glance

The primary period of the diet keeps going multi week. During the underlying three days, members are permitted to devour 1,000 calories as three sirtfood juices and one sirtfood-rich dinner, which can likewise join non-sirtfoods. During days four to seven, calories are expanded to 1,500 every day, and can incorporate two sirtfood juices and two sirtfood-rich suppers.

The subsequent stage keeps going 14 days, and it is during this time most weight loss allegedly happens regardless of a shift away from calorie limitation. The attention is currently on solidifying your new-gained sirtfood dietary patterns with three sirtfood-rich dinners and one green squeeze a day.

SIRTFOOD AND DISEASE

The investigation of maturing in invertebrate model creatures has delivered central new perceptions about instruments of eukaryotic maturing. Among the qualities that have been appeared to direct maturing in different species are SIR2 and its practical orthologs that make up a group of protein deacetylases named Sirtuins. It has been known for four decades that histones can be acetylated (Roth et al., 2001), despite the fact that the catalysts that acetylate and deacetylate lysine buildups on histones and different proteins have just been found all the more as of late. Histone and protein deacetylases fall into four classes with the yeast proteins Rpd3 (class I), Hda1 (class II), and Sir2 (class III) filling in as sanction individuals from the three significant classes (Blander and Guarente, 2004, Sengupta and Seto, 2004). Human HDAC11, the sole individual from class IV, is moderated in mice and D. melanogaster however not C. elegans and yeast (Gao et al., 2002). Class III deacetylases, the Sirtuins, are special in that they require NAD as a cofactor (Blander and Guarente, 2004, Denu, 2003). In an entangled two-advance response, Sirtuins couple lysine deacetylation to NAD hydrolysis, yielding O-acetyl-ADP-ribose and nicotinamide (Denu, 2003). All things considered, Sirtuin action might be constrained by cell [NAD]/[NADH] proportions and react to changes in cell digestion (Lin et al., 2000, Lin et al., 2002, Lin et al., 2004).

Both class I and III deacetylases have been connected to maturing (Bitterman et al., 2003), albeit most examinations have concentrated on the class III Sirtuins. Expanded Sir2 action has been accounted for to improve yeast replicative life range (depicted underneath) (Kaeberlein et al., 1999), just as the life length of C. elegans and D. melanogaster (Rogina and Helfand, 2004, Tissenbaum and Guarente, 2001). Conversely, decreased Sir2 action broadens yeast ordered life range (portrayed beneath) under supplement poor conditions or in blend with transformations in qualities, for example, RAS2 and SCH9, which work in glucose-responsive sign transduction pathways (Fabrizio et al., 2005). Various investigations of Sirtuin work have been acted in mammalian cells, in spite of the fact that it stays obscure whether Sirtuins legitimately control life length. Right now, analyze the job of Sir2 and different Sirtuins in invertebrate maturing. Also, we examine Sirtuin works in warm blooded creatures and how they may influence human life span and age-related sickness.

Sirtuins and Yeast Replicative Life Span

The topsy-turvy division normal for the yeast S. cerevisiae is the reason for replicative life-range estimations. Mother cells give ascend by maturing to littler, effectively recognizable girl cells. Micromanipulation is utilized to expel progressive little girls, which are considered ages and arranged (Mortimer and Johnston, 1959). Extensive exertion has been coordinated toward identifying qualities that direct yeast replicative maturing. Analysts have set accentuation on transformations and intercessions that lengthen yeast life range, thinking that mediations diminishing life length may not be straightforwardly connected to the maturing procedure. Until this point, around 50 changes, for the most part quality cancellations, have been accounted for to bring about expanded replicative life range (Bitterman et al., 2003, Kaeberlein et al., 2005b).

The principal interface among SIR2 and maturing originated from the finding that specific transformations in a segment of the yeast SIR complex brought about augmentation of replicative life range (Kennedy et al., 1995). At that point, the SIR complex (Sir2, Sir3, and Sir4) was known to curb interpretation of two yeast quiet mating-type loci (which contain untranscribed duplicates of mating assurance qualities) and of qualities put close to yeast telomeres (Rusche et al., 2003). At first, it was conjectured that SIR movement at telomeres might be managing yeast maturing, however follow-up examination demonstrated that improved life range corresponded with relocalization of the SIR complex to the nucleolus (Kennedy et al., 1997), the subnuclear area of ribosomal DNA (rDNA) qualities and a significant site of ribosome biogenesis.

Homologous recombination inside rDNA rehashes can prompt the development of extrachromosomal rDNA circles (ERCs). Sir2 hinders rDNA recombination and can likewise quell translation of embedded qualities that are interpreted by PolII (Rusche et al., 2003). Since ERCs contain a site of replication inception however no centromere, they experience replication during S stage yet stay in the mother cell core during mitosis. Aggregation of ERCs inside a mother cell is one reason for yeast replicative maturing (Sinclair and Guarente, 1997). Without SIR2, the pace of ERC arrangement is improved and cells are fleeting (Kaeberlein et al., 1999). Diminished recombination intervened by SIR2 overexpression or cancellation of the FOB1 quality prompts lower ERC levels and results in expanded yeast replicative life length (Defossez et al., 1999, Kaeberlein et al., 1999). Fob1 has replication fork blocking movement and furthermore advances recombination inside the rDNA (Kobayashi and Horiuchi, 1996). Albeit expanded movement of Sir2 orthologs is related with life-range expansion in worms and flies (Rogina and Helfand, 2004, Tissenbaum and Guarente, 2001), there is no proof of a connection among ERCs and maturing in any life form other than yeast.

Calorie Restriction and Yeast Replicative Aging

Calorie limitation (CR), characterized as a decrease in organismal vitality consumption, has been appeared to improve life span of creatures running from yeast to warm blooded animals. Yeast is a significant framework wherein to contemplate calorie limitation since supplement responsive pathways directing cell development are generally surely known. CR in yeast can be initiated by a decrease of glucose in the development media or by transformations, (for example, the erasure of hexokinase 2) that lessen the digestion of glucose (Lin et al., 2000). The job of Sir2 in the calorie limitation reaction is questionable (Guarente, 2005, Kennedy et al., 2005). Significantly, it stays undisputed that expanded Sir2 action prompts replicative life-range augmentation; just the proposed connection among Sir2 and CR has been raised doubt about.

At first, it was accounted for that SIR2 was required forever range augmentation by calorie limitation in yeast. This end depended on an additionally undisputed finding that brief strains lacking SIR2 didn't display life-length expansion under CR conditions. Without SIR2, ERCs aggregate. Along these lines, the finding that

CR neglects to expand life length in a strain lacking SIR2 can be deciphered in one of two different ways. Either CR legitimately prompts a decrease in ERC levels by improving Sir2 movement (Lin et al., 2000) or yeast strains lacking SIR2, which have an inexact half decrease in mean replicative life-length potential, rashly capitulate to raised ERCs and don't live long enough to react to CR.

It has been accounted for that CR causes hearty life-length expansion without SIR2 as long as ERCs are kept at low levels by erasure of FOB1 (Kaeberlein et al., 2004), a finding that has since been upheld by another gathering (Lamming et al., 2005) yet not bolstered in a previous investigation utilizing a different yeast strain foundation (Lin et al., 2002). This was deciphered by Kaeberlein et al. to demonstrate that SIR2 is required not as an immediate effector of calorie limitation however in a roundabout way to keep up low ERC levels and along these lines empower the cells to live long enough to react to CR (Kaeberlein et al., 2004). To repeat, there is general understanding that CR can expand replicative life range in a strain lacking both SIR2 and FOB1 however not in a strain that needs just SIR2. Be that as it may, follow-up examinations and translations thereof have driven different gatherings to different ends with respect to the significance of Sir2 for the CR reaction (see underneath). CR actualized by a decrease in amino acids is likewise answered to broaden yeast replicative life length (Jiang et al., 2002). Expansion right now free of SIR2.

One of the creators (B.K.K.) is at the focal point of the contest with respect to the significance of Sir2 in the CR reaction. Notwithstanding, we will exhibit the two perspectives as well as could be expected. The discussion as of now lays on the degree of glucose restriction used to actualize the CR reaction. Guarente, Lin, Sinclair, and partners accept that lessening the glucose fixation from 2% to 0.5% (4× decrease) is perfect since it minimally affects yeast development rate and might be all the more physiologically like degrees of calorie limitation utilized in other model life forms (Lamming et al., 2006, Lin and Guarente, 2006). They recommend that CR interceded by a decrease in glucose fixation to 0.05% might be SIR2 autonomous and intervened through a different system. Kaeberlein, Kennedy, and partners have to a great extent, however not only, utilized 0.05% glucose (40× decrease) since it amplifies life-length expansion (Kaeberlein et al., 2004, Kaeberlein et al., 2005a, Kaeberlein et al., 2006b), allowing simpler understanding of epistasis examination (Clancy et al., 2002). They bolster a model whereby life-range augmentation by CR is Sirtuin autonomous and not on a very basic level different at either level of glucose constraint (Kaeberlein et al., 2005a, Kaeberlein et al., 2006a, Kaeberlein et al., 2006b). At either 0.5% or 0.05% glucose, CR broadens life length in a way subject to the supplement responsive kinases, TOR, PKA, and SCH9 (the Akt ortholog) (see brief conversation underneath) (Fabrizio et al., 2001, Kaeberlein et al., 2005d, Lin et al., 2000). These supplement responsive kinases control various downstream reactions including ribosome biogenesis and cell development, stress reactions, and autophagy. Which of these are significant forever length augmentation stays to be resolved. Despite the fact that erasure of SCH9 reduces recombination in the rDNA (Prusty and Keil, 2004), it is obvious from an assortment of epistasis contemplates that this phenotype doesn't clarify replicative life-length augmentation. For instance, twofold freaks lacking both SCH9 and FOB1 endure any longer than freaks lacking just FOB1, which as of now have very low degrees of ERCs (Kaeberlein et al., 2005d).

Life-range expansion by CR at 0.5% or 0.05% glucose can happen without SIR2, as long as FOB1 is likewise erased (Kaeberlein et al., 2004, Lamming et al., 2005). Two discoveries drove Lamming et al. to recommend that different Sirtuins were, as one with Sir2, acting in an excess design to intercede the calorie limitation reaction under these conditions (Lamming et al., 2005). To start with, nicotinamide, a known inhibitor of Sirtuin enzymatic action, can hinder probably a portion of the life-length augmentation by CR even without Sir2 (Kaeberlein et al., 2005a, Lamming et al., 2005). Second, a screen for qualities that when overexpressed prompted upgraded rDNA hushing brought about the identification of HST2, another Sirtuin (Lamming et al., 2005). In spite of the fact that Hst2 is regularly cytoplasmic (Perrod et al., 2001), under CR conditions it is accounted for to relocalize to the core (Lamming et al., 2005). Further, Lamming et al. report that, comparably to strains lacking SIR2, yeast lacking just HST2 display raised rDNA recombination and a short life range. The discovering about rDNA recombination appears differently in relation to a past report by Gasser and associates, who found that a yeast strain lacking HST2 shows decreased rDNA recombination (Perrod et al., 2001).

At 0.5% glucose, Lamming et al. report that CR neglects to expand life range in a strain lacking both SIR2 and HST2, prompting the end that CR broadens life length by lessening rDNA recombination and ERC development in a SIR2-and HST2-subordinate design (Lamming et al., 2005). Hst1, another Sirtuin, may likewise make up for Sir2 in certain strains. Another gathering has discovered utilizing the equivalent hereditary foundation that CR broadens life range in yeast strains that need SIR2, HST2, and FOB1 or in yeast that additionally need HST1 (Kaeberlein et al., 2006b). The reason(s) for these divergent discoveries are as a rule effectively discussed (Kaeberlein et al., 2006b, Lamming et al., 2006).

At long last, life span expansion by CR has been connected to cell breath. Work from Guarente, Sinclair, and partners has prompted the model that CR prompts raised NAD levels (Lin et al., 2002), decreased NADH levels (Lin et al., 2004), as well as diminished nicotinamide levels (Anderson et al., 2003, Bitterman et al., 2002), which thus lead to Sir2 enactment. Decreasing glucose levels in yeast improves the respiratory pace of the facultative anaerobe, and it has been suggested this upgraded pace of breath prompts expanded [NAD]/[NADH] proportions. Besides, CR neglects to increment replicative life range of respiratory-insufficient yeast (Lin et al., 2002), although this finding has additionally been questioned (Kaeberlein et al., 2005a). Regardless of whether differential degrees of glucose hardship underlie the divergent discoveries of these examinations likewise keeps on being discussed (Kaeberlein et al., 2006a, Lin and Guarente, 2006).

Sir2 and Yeast Chronological Life Span

The ordered life-length models maturing in the common habitat since it is a proportion of the endurance of yeast populaces in a nondividing state (Longo et al., 1997). The middle sequential life length of S. cerevisiae wild-type DBY746 or SP1 yeast developed in glucose medium (SDC) is 6 to 7 days. Under these conditions wild-type DBY746 cells have overabundance ethanol accessible for vitality creation and keep up high metabolic rates for most of the life length. A type of serious calorie limitation, accomplished by changing cells from ethanol/glucose-containing medium to water between days 1 and 5, causes a reduction in metabolic rates and stretches out endurance by 2-to 3-overlay (Fabrizio et al., 2004a, Longo et al., 1997).

Yeast strains with decreased movement of Ras2 or any of the supplement responsive kinases Sch9, PKA, and TOR have broadened sequential life length (Fabrizio et al., 2001, Fabrizio et al., 2003, Fabrizio et al., 2004b, Powers et al., 2006). Significantly, Sch9 is a utilitarian homolog of Akt/PKB, a part of the moderated master maturing pathways of worms, flies, and mice (Longo and Finch, 2003).

As opposed to the job of ERCs in yeast replicative maturing, superoxide seems to assume a focal job in S. cerevisiae sequential maturing and demise. Truth be told, the superoxide-delicate 4Fe-4S group catalyst aconitase is inactivated going before the high mortality stage (Fabrizio et al., 2001), and overexpression of the superoxide dismutases SOD1 or SOD2 expands ordered life range (Fabrizio et al., 2003). Unconstrained DNA transformation recurrence likewise increments with sequential age, although its job in maturing and demise remains inadequately comprehended (Fabrizio et al., 2004a, Fabrizio et al., 2005).

The job of Sir2 in the ordered endurance of nondividing yeast cells has as of late been inspected (Fabrizio et al., 2005) and gives off an impression of being very different from its job in the yeast replicative life range. Cancellation of SIR2 expands pressure opposition yet has no impact on the sequential life length of wild-type yeast developed and kept up in medium. In any case, erasure of SIR2 expands further the ordered life length brought about by serious CR (hatching in water) (Fabrizio et al., 2005) or brought about by transformations that abatement PKA or Sch9 action. Besides, the overexpression of SIR2 has no impact on the ordered life length of wild-type cells and lessens the life range of cells lacking Sch9 action (Fabrizio et al., 2005). Different Sirtuins have not been analyzed right now. Proof exists for two potential components by which erasure of SIR2 brings about life-range augmentation when combined with diminished supplement responsive kinase action or CR. To start with, cancellation of SIR2 in blend with diminished PKA or Sch9 movement was found to build the statement of many pressure opposition and sporulation qualities and to diminish the pace of DNA transformations that amass with age in postmitotic conditions (Fabrizio et al., 2005). This stands out from the job of Sir2 in mitotically dynamic cells, where it advances genome security by curbing recombination (Blander and Guarente, 2004). Second, Fabrizio et al. report that cells lacking SIR2 have raised degrees of the liquor dehydrogenase Adh2 (Fabrizio et al., 2005). Mitotically dynamic yeast cells fundamentally create vitality through aging, which prompts the generation of ethanol. As fermentable carbon sources become rare and ethanol aggregates, yeast experience a metabolic shift and start to use ethanol as a vitality source, just entering stationary stage after ethanol levels are generally exhausted. Without Sir2, expanded liquor dehydrogenase action prompts increasingly quick ethanol debasement and section into a progressively steady postmitotic state. The component by which Sir2 contrarily manages Adh2 levels as cells enter a postmitotic state is yet to be resolved. Expanded ethanol take-up may speak to an endeavor by cells lacking SIR2 to get ready for extensive stretches of starvation.

In rundown, even though the cancellation of SIR2 diminishes and its overexpression expands the yeast replicative life range, changing Sir2 levels doesn't significantly influence the sequential life length. In any case, when joined with serious CR-or life-length expanding changes that diminish the movement of the Ras and Sch9 pathways, transformations in SIR2 do broaden the ordered life range and Sir2 overexpression limits life-length expansion in freaks lacking SCH9. Loss of SIR2 may advance passage into an express that secures cells against maturing during starvation. These outcomes propose that Sir2 assumes totally different jobs in the guideline of replicative and sequential life range.

One Model Organism, Two Measures of Aging?

The replicative life length of yeast is in numerous regards like the replicative life range of mammalian fibroblasts and lymphocytes, which experience a set number of populace doublings in culture. Along these lines, replicative maturing in yeast might be a model to consider replicative maturing in mitotically dynamic mammalian cells. Paradoxically, sequential maturing in yeast may serve to display maturing in postmitotic mammalian cells (e.g., neurons) and living beings. Whatever degree do comparative pathways control the systems that lead to replicative and ordered maturing in a similar model living being?

Though prior investigations demonstrated likenesses yet additionally significant differences between the guideline of replicative and ordered life range, later examinations are starting to recommend that there might be just one type of "maturing" in S. cerevisiae with two different ways to quantify it. An enormous scale scan for freaks with an all-inclusive replicative life length prompted the identification of erasure freaks in sch9 and tor1, additionally ensnared in ordered life-range expansion (Fabrizio et al., 2001, Kaeberlein et al., 2005d, Powers et al., 2006). In this manner, supplement responsive kinases control maturing of both mitotic and postmitotic cells. Regardless of whether the effectors that controls each sort of maturing downstream of these kinases are a similar stay to be resolved.

Strikingly, diminished movement of orthologs of these kinases as well as of the pathways where they work lead to life-range expansion in worms, flies, and warm-blooded creatures (Kenyon, 2005, Longo and Finch, 2003). We presume that hindrance of these supplement responsive kinases prompts life-length augmentation in warm blooded creatures since it gives particular, helpful impacts in both mitotic and postmitotic populaces of cells. Backing for this originates from yeast replicative and sequential life-range considers yet in addition from life span tests in C. elegans, where it was indicated that diminished insulin/IGF-1 flagging can slow an assortment of age-related phenotypes in particular tissues (Garigan et al., 2002). Comparable impacts have been watched for CR in mice.

For yeast replicative life range, twofold freaks lacking FOB1 and either SCH9 or TOR1 are very seemingly perpetual, proposing that the collection of ERCs brought about by Fob1 may, to a certain extent, veil the impact of loss of SCH9 or TOR1 on replicative life-length augmentation. Hence, ERCs might be liable for one error between the impact of Sir2 on replicative and sequential life range. If Sir2 is missing, ERCs aggregate early and either execute the cell or forestall its division. If Sir2 is overexpressed, ERC levels are diminished and replicative life range is upgraded. ERCs may then be seen as an operator that hurries demise specifically in yeast and clouds other progressively widespread maturing forms. Be that as it may, cancellation of SIR2 doesn't expand the replicative life range of strains lacking SCH9 or TOR1 even without FOB1, so there must be other fundamental differences also.

The power of common choice against the presence of "abandons" is extremely high in youthful living beings, yet it decreases at cutting edge ages. Yeast mother cells don't have to create 25 girls to guarantee state endurance or even a maximal settlement development rate, and, therefore, injurious occasions that are specific to old mother cells, (for example, ERC arrangement or diminished development rates) may not be dependent upon counter-selection. Along these lines, ERCs seem, by all accounts, to be a significant reason for maturing just in yeast exposed to conditions not ordinarily experienced in indigenous habitats. Conversely, different instruments of maturing might be moderated, and proof not just from yeast ordered and replicative maturing examines, yet in addition from higher eukaryotes, is starting to show that the Sch9 (Akt), Ras, and Tor might be all inclusive controllers of these systems. Sir2 is obviously significant forever length guideline however it might play either an ace or an enemy of maturing job in different life forms relying upon the accessibility of supplements and on the movement of glucose flagging pathways.

Sir2 and Aging in Other Invertebrates

Two other model life forms where maturing has been contemplated broadly are C. elegans and D. melanogaster. Right now condense discoveries with respect to the job of Sir2 orthologs in maturing in these spineless creatures. Different Sirtuins are available in the two life forms, yet their jobs in maturing have not been learned. In C. elegans, expanded measurement of the SIR2 ortholog, sir-2.1, builds the mean life range by up to half (Tissenbaum and Guarente, 2001), and this augmentation requires the FOXO translation factor DAF-16, which is known to be controlled by the insulin/IGF-1 pathway. Instead of acting legitimately in the insulin/IGF-1 flagging pathway, two late investigations recommend that SIR-2.1 may act in an equal pathway that unites at the purpose of DAF-16 guideline (Wang et al., 2006) (Berdichevsky et al., 2006). In the two examinations, both C. elegans 14-3-3 proteins were identified as SIR-2.1 interactors, a fascinating discovering on the grounds that mammalian 14-3-3 proteins are known to tie FOXO translation factors and sequester them in the cytoplasm (Brunet et al., 1999). In spite of the fact that life-length expansion by SIR-2.1 overexpression can be obstructed by lessening articulation of 14-3-3 proteins, this isn't the situation for transformations that upset the insulin pathway (Wang et al., 2006) (Berdichevsky et al., 2006). For example, the long life length of a daf-2 freak isn't influenced by a decrease in 14-3-3. Indeed, erasure of sir-2.1 doesn't decrease the life range of a daf-2 freak and rather appears to somewhat expand it, steady with the more extended ordered life length watched for yeast lacking both SIR2 and the Akt homolog SCH9 (Berdichevsky et al., 2006, Fabrizio et al., 2005, Wang and Tissenbaum, 2006).

Berdichevsky et al. suggest that SIR-2.1 is a piece of a pressure reaction pathway that manages DAF-16 action in a way reliant on 14-3-3 proteins (Berdichevsky et al., 2006). Steady with this thought, an invalid freak of C. elegans sir-2.1 has a somewhat shorter life length as well as shows affectability to an assortment of stresses including hydrogen peroxide, UV light, and warmth stun (Wang and Tissenbaum, 2006). These outcomes just incompletely concur with those watched for nondividing yeast. Truth be told, in yeast lacking SIR2 the ordered life range is either ordinary or somewhat shorter, DNA transformations are progressively visit, yet affectability to warm stun and oxidative pressure is diminished (Fabrizio et al., 2005). SIR-2.1 is likewise answered to be significant for hushing of transgenes embedded into genomic rehash components, maybe in a way practically equivalent to Sir2-subordinate quieting in yeast (Jedrusik and Schulze, 2003). Regardless of whether this action is significant for life span guideline stays to be resolved.

Different measures have been proposed for calorie limitation in C. elegans, including utilization of eat-2 freaks that eat not exactly wild-type worms, development in axenic media that comes up short on a bacterial nourishment source, and decreased presentation to nourishment source or dietary limitation (Walker et al., 2005). The reliance of sir-2.1 has been resolved for eat-2 freaks and dietary limitation, with to some degree different outcomes. Life-length augmentation by eat-2 freaks is halfway smothered by cancellation of sir-2.1 (Wang and Tissenbaum, 2006). Interestingly, life-length expansion by dietary limitation isn't influenced by sir-2.1 cancellation (M. Kaeberlein, individual correspondence). Likewise, while life-range expansion by sir-2.1 overexpression is daf-16 ward (Tissenbaum and Guarente, 2001), life-length augmentation by CR isn't (Lakowski and Hekimi, 1998).

Little atom activators and inhibitors of Sirtuins have been accounted for. Resveratrol has been proposed as a little atom agonist of yeast Sir2 and of its orthologs in worms, flies, and vertebrates and has been examined with regards to life span (Wood et al., 2004). Resveratrol was identified in a screen for Sirtuin activators utilizing a nonbiological substrate reasonable for high-throughput fluorescent examination (Howitz et al., 2003). In any case, different gatherings have demonstrated that the stimulatory impacts of resveratrol on Sirtuin catalyst enactment are specific to this nonnative substrate (Borra et al., 2005, Kaeberlein et al., 2005c). No improvement of catalyst movement was seen with local acetylated peptides. One plausibility is that resveratrol just invigorates Sirtuin movement toward specific substrates in vivo. On the other hand, the impacts of reseveratrol might be to a great extent Sirtuin autonomous, an attestation predictable with perceptions that the polyphenol compound has a plenty of different exercises. Reports strife about whether resveratrol broadens yeast life range (Howitz et al., 2003, Kaeberlein et al., 2005c).

In C. elegans, sir-2.1-subordinate life-length expansion has been watched for resveratrol (Wood et al., 2004). An ongoing report anyway has recommended that, as opposed to upgrade SIR-2.1 action in worms, resveratrol may expand life range by alienating it (Viswanathan et al., 2005). Likewise, not at all like sir-2.1 overexpression, resveratrol expands life length in a daf-16-autonomous way. The key objective forever length expansion due to resveretrol treatment seems, by all accounts, to be abu-11, an endoplasmic reticulum (ER) stress-family quality. Either expansion of resveratrol or, inquisitively, sir-2.1 cancellation prompts upgraded abu-11 articulation, which is thusly required forever length augmentation. The creators set forth a model to clarify these apparently confusing discoveries by suggesting that (1) resveratrol may tie to SIR-2.1 and change its specificity toward substrates to such an extent that deacetylation of certain substrates might be upgraded while deacetylation of different substrates is hindered and (2) SIR-2.1 has numerous capacities that encroach on life span guideline with the net impact being that overexpression expands life length. Subsequently, as with Sir2 in yeast, SIR-2.1 in worms may have a few exercises that advance life span and others that breaking point it. Maybe the most intriguing finding from this investigation is that overexpression of abu-11 expands worm life length, ensnaring ER worry as a constraining variable in worm life span.

In flies, the Sir2 ortholog dSir2 has been accounted for to expand life range also (Rogina and Helfand, 2004). What's more, life-length augmentation by CR is obstructed in strains lacking dSir2. These discoveries propose that CR works through a Sir2-subordinate system right now. Freak flies with diminished Rpd3 (class I deacetylase) movement show expanded life length that is subject to dSir2, demonstrating that the two deacetylases are in a solitary pathway managing maturing with Rpd3 upstream (Rogina and Helfand, 2004, Rogina et al., 2002). It has not been resolved whether Rpd3 directs [NAD]/[NADH] proportions in flies. Life-range augmentation by resveratrol is likewise answered to be dSir2 subordinate (Wood et al., 2004). Little is thought about dSir2 work in flies, particularly with respect to maturing specific capacities. This deacetylase has been accounted for to be engaged with transcriptional restraint (Newman et al., 2002), at any rate to some extent through communications with Hairy, a translation calculates included formative guideline (Rosenberg and Parkhurst, 2002). Regardless of whether dSir2 manages the insulin pathway in flies stays to be resolved.

In outline, overexpression of Sir2 orthologs builds fly and worm life range, and the connections between Sir2 orthologs and calorie limitation seem conflicting among living beings and stay to be completely comprehended. It appears to be incomprehensible that the catalyst for analyzing the life range of worms and flies overexpressing their Sir2 orthologs got from yeast replicative maturing contemplates, given that the proposed job of Sir2 in life span guideline, lessening ERC generation, appears not to be preserved. We offer three potential clarifications to determine this conundrum. Initially, Sir2 in yeast may have different capacities beside decreased ERC creation that advance replicative life span, and this movement might be rationed. Second, worm and fly Sir2 orthologs may expand life length by stifling recombination at other chromosomal areas that are increasingly delicate (e.g., dreary DNA) and that don't exist in yeast or impact yeast life range. It is difficult to decipher this model with regards to C. elegans where daf-16 is required for the life span impacts of sir-2.1 overexpression. At last, Sir2 orthologs may have developed to couple metabolic signs to specific life span upgrading capacities in different living beings, a model advanced by Guarente and associates (Guarente and Picard, 2005). How this last model would fit with developmental hypotheses of maturing stays to be settled. We should anticipate further trials in every one of these life forms to start to differentiate between these models or devise a different one. Further adding to the disjointedness is the finding that loss of SIR2 in certain settings improves yeast ordered life length and that its overexpression doesn't influence or lessens sequential life span (Fabrizio et al., 2005).

Sirtuins in Mammals

The maturing phenotype of mice overexpressing Sirt1, and the impacts of CR on life span in a mouse lacking Sirt1, has not yet been resolved. Albeit a dominant part of Sirt1 invalid creatures surrender to formative deformities during early postnatal improvement (Cheng et al., 2003, McBurney et al., 2003), the rest of the mice endure and have phenotypes looking like mice overexpressing IGFBP-1 or lacking IGF-I (Longo and Finch, 2003) (see beneath). In Sirt1-insufficient grown-up survivors, Chen et al. report that calorie limitation neglects to prompt expanded physical movement (Chen et al., 2005a), a typical CR-initiated conduct change in wild-type mice. Be that as it may, physiologic changes like those brought about by CR, for example, decreased blood glucose, triglycerides, and insulin levels, happen ordinarily in these creatures. Even though these last phenotypes may be relied upon to broaden life span, the impact of Sirt1 inadequacy alone or in blend with CR stays to be set up. By and by, various investigations have announced in well evolved creatures interesting elements of Sirtuins that may relate to maturing. In the accompanying segments, we layout a portion of these discoveries, concentrating on results that identify with maturing and age-related malady.

Sir2/Sirt1, Genomic Instability, and Oncogenesis

Starting connections between Sir2 work and the reaction to DNA harm originated from considers in S. cerevisiae. In proliferating yeast, a few reports demonstrate that Sir2 ensures against DNA harm by inciting nonhomologous end joining and homologous recombination pathways, a capacity which seems to rely upon the derepression of quiet mating-type qualities (Fabrizio et al., 2005, Lee et al., 1999). Sir2 likewise intercedes the deviated legacy of oxidatively harmed proteins during cell division (Aguilaniu et al., 2003). Mother cells have a constrained life length, however the provinces they produce will keep proliferating as long as adequate supplements are accessible. This hilter kilter legacy limits harmed proteins to the mother cell, likely guaranteeing the age of moderately harm free little girls and proceeded with state proliferation. Interestingly, Sir2 seems to advance ordered age-subordinate genomic unsteadiness in extensive freaks. S. cerevisiae cells aggregate unconstrained DNA transformations with ordered age, and this gathering is radically diminished in strains lacking both SCH9 and SIR2 (Fabrizio et al., 2005). In spite of the fact that this impact of Sir2 insufficiency gives off an impression of being autonomous of the derepression of quiet mating-type qualities, the instruments by which Sir2 advances age-subordinate genomic flimsiness are not known.

In warm blooded creatures, extensive proof exists to recommend that the tumor silencer p53 is an objective for deacetylation by Sirt1 (Cheng et al., 2003). Under typical cell conditions for proliferation, p53, a transcriptional activator, is exceptionally precarious (Gu et al., 2004). p53 adjustment happens as a major aspect of a checkpoint reaction to cell stress (counting DNA harm) and results in proliferative capture, trailed by either reemergence into the cell cycle, senescence, or apoptosis. Acetylation of p53 prompts improved transcriptional enactment as a major aspect of the checkpoint reaction. By deacetylating p53, Sirt1 may kill p53 after recuperation from worry to permit cell proliferation to continue. Even though it has been indicated that expanded Sirt1 movement prompts hypoacetylation of p53 and constraint of p53 target qualities (Luo et al., 2001, Vaziri et al., 2001), the cell outcomes of this stay being referred to. While Sirt1 movement was initially answered to hinder apoptosis through deacetylation of p53 (Langley et al., 2002, Luo et al., 2001), later reports propose that despite the fact that Sirt1 can deacetylate p53 there is little impact on p53-interceded organic results (Kamel et al., 2006, Solomon et al., 2006). Different pressure reaction related proteins connected to Sirt1 are Ku70 and NF-κB (see underneath) (Cohen et al., 2004, Yeung et al., 2004). Ku70, a DNA fix factor, is accounted for to be an objective for deacetylation by Sirt1, which is another instrument by which Sirt1 may repress cell demise (Cohen et al., 2004).

Developing connections between Sir.2-1 and daf-16 in worms, a few examinations have tried the theory that Sirt1 can manage mammalian FOXO translation factors through direct authoritative or potentially deacetylation. Sirt1 deacetylation can either prompt actuation or constraint of FOXO-subordinate interpretation relying upon the unique situation (Greer and Brunet, 2005). Current reasoning is that deacetylation of FOXO factors by Sirt1 may prompt enactment of a lot of pressure safe variables, influencing the equalization toward stress opposition and away from apoptosis (Brunet et al., 2004). There additionally exists a mind boggling interchange between FOXOs, Sirt1, and p53, with each having the option to direct the other two in probably some cell settings (Greer and Brunet, 2005). Since every one of the three of these proteins have been connected to maturing, it is basic that future investigations outline these mind boggling cooperations.

Sirt1 work has likewise been inspected with regards to cell senescence in cell culture. Chua et al. report that mouse undeveloped organism fibroblasts lacking Sirt1 are impervious to senescence within the sight of sublethal, incessant oxidative pressure (Chua et al., 2005). Strangely, oncogene-instigated senescence happens ordinarily in these cells. Reliable with this outcome, nicotinamide, a sirtuin inhibitor, has been accounted for in another examination to expand the replicative life range of essential human fibroblasts (Lim et al., 2006), albeit no trials were exhibited that straightforwardly connect the activities of nicotinamide to Sirt1 or different Sirtuins right now. Primer investigations inspecting joins between Sirt1 capacity and malignant growth recommend that it is improved Sirt1 movement that might be oncogenic. For example, treatment of human bosom and lung malignancy cells with Sirtinol, another Sirt1 inhibitor, has been found to prompt a senescent-like development capture (Ota et al., 2006). Related discoveries were accounted for by Ford et al. (Portage et al., 2005), who utilized RNAi to quiet articulation of Sirt1. Right now, decrease of Sirt1 prompted development capture as well as apoptosis in human epithelial malignant growth lines yet not essential epithelial cells.

Inhibitors of class I and class II histone deacetylases are under clinical preliminaries as chemotherapeutic specialists. The antitumor impacts of these inhibitors likely originate from their capacity to reactivate translation of tumor silencer qualities in blend with DNA-demethylating operators. A comparable job has as of late been proposed for the Sirt1 inhibitors, which were found to advance the reactivation of tumor silencer quality interpretation in human bosom and colon malignant growth lines (Pruitt et al., 2006). Right now, articulation could be accomplished without inhibitors of DNA methylation despite the fact that the advertisers being referred to remained exceptionally methylated. Although there is no broad understanding concerning the systems by which Sirt1 may advance oncogenesis, these examinations by and large point to the requirement for additional examination and the potential job of Sirtuin inhibitors in disease treatment. These outcomes might be reliable with the impact of SIR2 cancellation transformations in expanding protection from oxidative harm, decreasing DNA harm, and broadening the yeast ordered life length in mix with changes in supplement responsive kinases (Fabrizio et al., 2005). In this way, both yeast Sir2 and mammalian Sirt1 can advance DNA harm or oncogenesis, even though they likewise assume significant jobs in ensuring against harm during cell development and organismal improvement.

Less firmly identified with the different Sirtuins, the essential movement of Sirt6 is ADP-ribosylation instead of deacetylation (Liszt et al., 2005). An ongoing report finds that mice lacking Sirt6 display upgraded genome precariousness prompting a wide scope of chromosomal inconsistencies just as phenotypes looking like untimely maturing, including cachexia, kyphosis, and osteopenia (Mostoslavsky et al., 2006). Numerous different changes prompting progeria in well evolved creatures are related with genome shakiness. Mostoslavsky et al. find that mice lacking Sirt6 have a scope of sensitivities to DNA-harming operators including MMS and ionizing radiation that are steady with absconds in base extraction fix (Mostoslavsky et al., 2006). The specific job of Sirt6 right now stays to be resolved.

Sirtuins and Mammalian Metabolism

Diminished insulin/IGF-I flagging is personally connected to improved life span in worms, flies, and mice (Longo and Finch, 2003). Further, cancellation of the yeast orthologs of Akt and Ras, which work downstream of mammalian insulin/IGF-I, brings about broadened replicative and sequential life length in yeast (Fabrizio et al., 2001, Fabrizio et al., 2003, Fabrizio et al., 2004b, Lin et al., 2000). Since insulin flagging connections extracellular glucose levels to cell digestion, and expanded life length in worms overexpressing sir-2.1 is reliant on daf-16, extensive exertion has been given to revealing the associations between Sirt1 capacity and digestion in well evolved creatures. Until this point in time, the aftereffects of these examinations have not created an away from of the job of Sirt1 in these procedures.

Two examinations have analyzed the capacity of Sirt1 in the arrival of insulin by pancreatic β cells. Bordone et al. revealed that a siRNA-upheld decrease of Sirt1 articulation in β cell lines prompts an expansion in the statement of uncoupling protein 2 (UCP2) and a decrease in insulin emission (Bordone et al., 2006). This finding may phenocopy nourishment hardship, which is known to actuate UCP2 articulation and diminish insulin discharge. In a subsequent report, Sirt1 articulation was raised specifically in the mouse pancreas, prompting decreased UCP2 articulation and upgraded insulin discharge during glucose incitement (Moynihan et al., 2005). Sirt1 additionally initiates gluconeogenic qualities and hepatic glucose yield through the transcriptional coactivator PGC-1 α (Rodgers et al., 2005). At any rate as to β cell work, decreased Sirt1 may impersonate as opposed to hinder the impacts of either CR or low-plasma IGF-I, in concurrence with different phenotypes portrayed underneath for Sirt1 invalid mice, including little body size and expanded degrees of IGFBP-1.

Sirtuins additionally have works in fat tissue. For example, Picard et al. show that Sirt1 advances fat activation in mammalian adipocytes by stifling PPARγ (Picard et al., 2004), and decreased fat substance has been connected to expanded life span (Bluher et al., 2003). Nonetheless, it is capacity and not the preparation of fat that has been reliably connected with life span expansion in worms, flies, and mice, evidently as a feature of a program planned for enduring extensive stretches of starvation (Longo and Finch, 2003). Remarkably Sirt3, a mitochondrial Sirtuin, is communicated to a great extent in darker fat, proposing a job for this deacetylase in versatile thermogenesis (Shi et al., 2005). Connections among maturing and Sirt3 presently can't seem to be accounted for.

Are the metabolic outcomes of adjusting Sirt1 levels professional or against maturing (or both)? Raised Sirt1 articulation may broaden life range by diminishing fat stockpiling. Then again, decreased Sirt1 levels cause changes undifferentiated from those saw in the enduring IGF-I-insufficient mice (McBurney et al., 2003). The job for Sirt1 in decreasing the statement of the IGF restricting protein, IGFBP-1, in expanding hepatic glucose yield, in expanding pancreatic insulin discharge, in activating fat, and in forestalling a smaller person phenotype raises the likelihood that Sirt1 may play both a master and hostile to maturing job in warm blooded creatures as has been appeared in S. cerevisiae, C. elegans, and mammalian cells (Fabrizio et al., 2005, Kaeberlein et al., 1999).

It will be imperative to decide if the job of Sirt1 in diminishing IGFBP-1 and fat stockpiling and expanding hepatic glucose yield and pancreatic insulin emission is proof for passage into a genius maturing mode and additionally whether Sirt1 controls frameworks that may advance physical action during times of starvation to discover nourishment or staying away from predation. Truth be told, the expansion in movement of mice during CR requires Sirt1 (Chen et al., 2005a). One plausibility is that, during CR, mammalian Sirt1 assumes a job in hindering section into a nonreproductive and decreased physical movement stage that might be portrayed by a more slow maturing rate (McBurney et al., 2003, Chen et al., 2005a), as appeared for the job of Sir2 in the S. cerevisiae sequential life range (Fabrizio et al., 2005).

Sirtuins and Neuro-degeneration

Both in C. elegans and well evolved creatures, specific neurological capacities have been ascribed to Sir2 orthologs. To consider neuronal cytotixicity in worms, Parker et al. built up a framework in which a part of the human Huntington infection related protein, htt, is communicated in contact receptor neurons (Parker et al., 2005). Either expanded measurements of sir-2.1 or introduction to resveratrol saved neuronal brokenness. The creators conjectured that SIR-2.1-subordinate enactment of stress-responsive daf-16 targets might be advancing cell endurance. Nothing to date has been accounted for that straightforwardly connects Sirt1 with htt in warm blooded creatures. Be that as it may, Sirt1 appears to repress axonal degeneration, a procedure that often goes before neuronal passing in neurodegenerative infections, for example, Parkinson's and Alzheimer's (Araki et al., 2004). This action of Sirt1 was found because moderate axonal degeneration in a strain of freak mice was connected to overexpression of a NAD biosynthetic compound. Of note, another exquisite investigation looking at axonal degeneration credited the advantages of expanded NAD biosynthesis to Sirt1-free modifications in neighborhood bioenergetics (Wang et al., 2005). These creators pinpointed the deteriorative decrease in NAD levels to axons and not the core where Sirt1 action is probably managed. A last report identified with neurodegeneration analyzed NF-κB motioning in microglia, an action connected to amyloid-β neuronal demise and Alzheimer's ailment, finding that overexpression of Sirt1 curbed NF-κB motioning by lessening RelA/p65 acetylation (Chen et al., 2005b). Together, these discoveries call for expanded assessment of Sirt1 as a potential defensive operator in neurons.

Sir2 Deacetylases: Anti-maturing, Pro-maturing, or Both?

In outline, the outcomes in S. cerevisiae and invertebrate model frameworks, combined with likenesses between Sirt1-insufficient and extensive IGF-I-lacking smaller person mice (Longo and Finch, 2003), propose that the most secure wager now is that Sir2 deacetylases play both ace and hostile to maturing jobs in different settings. One speculation to be tried is that decreased Sir2/Sirt1 movement can advance life-range expansion by causing section into a moderate maturing starvation reaction stage though Sir2/Sirt1 overexpression can advance life-length augmentation by actuating different changes, for example, fat breakdown and improved physical action.

The field basically anticipates investigations of mouse life span. Will mice overexpressing Sirt1, mice insufficient in Sirt1, or neither appreciate broadened life span? Will CR expand life length in mice lacking Sirt1? Will Sirt1 lack further expand the life range of mice with transformations in the IGF-1/Akt pathway? Other basic robotic inquiries additionally stay to be replied. What are the key focuses of the Sirt1 deacetylase? Does resveratrol invigorate Sirtuin action toward natural substrates and, if things being what they are, which ones? These outcomes and others will no uncertainty start to clarify the connections among Sirtuins and mammalian life span.

Over the previous decade, MIT researcher Leonard Guarente '74 and others have indicated that low-calorie diets incite a complete physiological reaction that advances endurance, all arranged by a lot of proteins called sirtuins.

Presently, Guarente and partners have indicated that sirtuins are additionally liable to assume a key job in the mental reaction to dietary limitation. When sirtuins are raised in the cerebrum, as happens when nourishment admission is cut, serotonin levels drop in mice and the creatures become substantially more on edge. Besides, in two huge hereditary investigations of people, the group found that changes that lift creation of sirtuins are usually connected with higher paces of nervousness and frenzy issue.

The specialists accept this nervousness might be a developmental adjustment that makes creatures—including people—increasingly careful under the pressure of scavenging all the more broadly for rare nourishment.

"It bodes well, in light of the fact that social impacts would be as versatile, and as chose by advancement, as physiological impacts," says -Guarente, an educator of science. "I don't believe it's amazing that conduct truly falls under the umbrella of common choice."

Guarente found around 20 years back that sirtuins drag out life range in yeast; from that point forward, they have been appeared to have comparative impacts in worms, mice, and different creatures. Ordinarily turned on considering stresses, for example, starvation or aggravation, the mixes coordinate an assortment of hormonal networks, administrative proteins, and qualities, with a net impact of keeping cells alive and solid.

His new research, distributed online in Cell in December, inspected mice with raised degrees of the SIRT1 protein in their cerebrums and mice with no SIRT1. Scientists set them on a round raised stage with two quadrants secured by a divider and two unprotected quadrants. "Ordinary mice will invest a lot of energy wandering out into the unprotected district, and super-restless mice will in general remain in the ensured zone," Guarente says.

The mice with extremely high sirtuin levels invested substantially more energy closer to the dividers, proposing that they were progressively restless. Mice lacking sirtuin were considerably bolder.

The group researched the cell instrument behind this wonder. They found that sirtuins help control levels of the synapse serotonin, since quite a while ago known to be basic for state of mind guideline.

The new research recommends that nervousness could be treated with drugs that hinder sirtuins. Be that as it may, it additionally offers purpose behind alert when treating patients with drugs that initiate sirtuins, a few of which are presently in clinical preliminaries for diabetes and other metabolic ailments. Those medications can't enter the cerebrum, however a few specialists are investigating the probability of utilizing sirtuin activators to treat neurological issue, for example, Alzheimer's malady. If such medications were created and affirmed, specialists may need to look for tension as a potential symptom.

"We need to learn as much as we can about the science of sirtuins, to illuminate the utilization regarding sirtuin medications to treat ailments," Guarente says. "The more we think about the science, the better position we'll be in to realize how to utilize the medications, how to portion them, and how to envision any conceivable symptoms."

SUPERFOODS

Healthfully, there is nothing of the sort as a superfood.

The term was instituted for showcasing purposes to impact nourishment patterns and sell items.

The nourishment business offers the superfood name on supplement rich food sources with an alleged ability to decidedly influence wellbeing.

Even though numerous nourishments could be depicted as super, it's imperative to comprehend that there is no single nourishment that holds the way to great wellbeing or infection counteraction.

Be that as it may, since the expression "superfood" doesn't appear to be going anyplace at any point soon, it might merit investigating some sound alternatives.

Here are 16 nourishments that might be deserving of the regarded superfood title.

1. Dim Leafy Greens

Dim green verdant vegetables (DGLVs) are a magnificent wellspring of supplements including folate, zinc, calcium, iron, magnesium, nutrient C and fiber.

Some portion of what makes DGLVs so super is their capability to diminish your danger of ceaseless sicknesses including coronary illness and type 2 diabetes.

They likewise contain significant levels of mitigating mixes known as carotenoids, which may ensure against particular sorts of malignant growth.

Some notable DGLVs include:

- Kale
- Swiss chard
- Collard greens

- Turnip greens

- Spinach

Some DGLVs have a harsh taste and not every person appreciates them plain. You can get imaginative by remembering them for your preferred soups, servings of mixed greens, smoothies, sautés and curries.

Synopsis

Dull green verdant vegetables are brimming with fiber and supplements which might be instrumental in forestalling certain incessant illnesses.

2. Berries

Berries are a healthful powerhouse of nutrients, minerals, fiber and cell reinforcements.

The solid cell reinforcement limit of berries is related with a diminished danger of coronary illness, malignant growth and other incendiary conditions.

Berries may likewise be successful in treating different stomach related and resistant related issue when utilized close by conventional medicinal treatments.

Probably the most widely recognized berries include:

- Raspberries

- Strawberries

- Blueberries

- Blackberries

- Cranberries

Regardless of whether you appreciate them as a component of your morning meal, as a treat, on a plate of mixed greens or in a smoothie, the medical advantages of berries are as flexible as their culinary applications.

Outline

Berries are loaded with supplements and cell reinforcements which may forestall certain illnesses and improve absorption.

3. Green Tea

Initially from China, green tea is a delicately jazzed refreshment with a wide exhibit of restorative properties.

Green tea is wealthy in cancer prevention agents and polyphenolic mixes which have solid mitigating impacts. One of the most common cell reinforcements in green tea is the catechin epigallocatechin gallate, or EGCG.

EGCG is likely what gives green tea its clear capacity to ensure against ceaseless sicknesses including coronary illness, diabetes and disease.

Research likewise demonstrates that the blend of catechins and caffeine in green tea may make it a viable instrument for weight loss in certain individuals.

Rundown

Green tea is cell reinforcement rich with numerous medical advantages including conceivable malignant growth avoidance.

4. Eggs

Eggs have truly been a disputable point in the nourishment world because of their elevated cholesterol content, yet they stay perhaps the most advantageous nourishment.

Entire eggs are plentiful in numerous supplements including B nutrients, choline, selenium, nutrient An, iron and phosphorus.

They're additionally stacked with top notch protein.

Eggs contain two strong cancer prevention agents, zeaxanthin and lutein, which are known to ensure vision and eye wellbeing.

In spite of fears encompassing egg utilization and elevated cholesterol, investigate demonstrates no quantifiable increment in coronary illness or diabetes hazard from eating up to 6–12 eggs for each week.

Truth be told, eating eggs could expand "great" HDL cholesterol in certain individuals, which may prompt a good decrease in coronary illness hazard. More research is expected to reach a distinct determination.

Rundown

Eggs are wealthy in great protein and one of a kind cancer prevention agents. Research demonstrates that eating eggs normally won't expand your danger of coronary illness or diabetes.

5. Vegetables

Vegetables, or heartbeats, are a class of plant nourishments made up of beans (counting soy), lentils, peas, peanuts and horse feed.

They procure the superfood mark since they're stacked with supplements and assume a job in forestalling and overseeing different maladies.

Vegetables are a rich wellspring of B nutrients, different minerals, protein and fiber.

Research shows that they offer numerous medical advantages including improved sort 2 diabetes the board, just as decreased circulatory strain and cholesterol.

Eating beans and vegetables routinely may likewise advance sound weight support, because of their capacity to improve sentiments of completion.

Outline

Vegetables are plentiful in numerous nutrients, protein and fiber. They may forestall some constant infections and bolster weight loss.

6. Nuts and Seeds

Nuts and seeds are wealthy in fiber, veggie lover protein and heart-solid fats.

They additionally pack different plant mixes with calming and cell reinforcement properties, which can secure against oxidative pressure.

Research shows that eating nuts and seeds can have a defensive impact against coronary illness.

Basic nuts and seeds include:

Almonds, walnuts, pistachios, pecans, cashews, Brazil nuts, macadamia nuts.

Peanuts — in fact a vegetable, yet often thought to be a nut.

Sunflower seeds, pumpkin seeds, chia seeds, flaxseeds, hemp seeds.

Strikingly, despite the fact that nuts and seeds are calorically thick, a few kinds of nuts are connected to weight loss when remembered for a decent diet.

Rundown

Nuts and seeds are brimming with fiber and heart-sound fats. They may lessen your danger of coronary illness and bolster weight loss.

7. Kefir (And Yogurt)

Kefir is a matured drink generally produced using milk that contains protein, calcium, B nutrients, potassium and probiotics.

Kefir is like yogurt yet has a slenderer consistency and regularly more probiotic strains than yogurt.

Aged, probiotic-rich nourishments like kefir have a few related medical advantages, including decreased cholesterol, brought down pulse, improved absorption and calming impacts.

Even though kefir is generally produced using dairy animals' milk, it's ordinarily all around endured by individuals with lactose prejudice because of the maturation of the lactose by microscopic organisms.

Nonetheless, it's likewise produced using non-dairy drinks, for example, coconut milk, rice milk and coconut water.

You can buy kefir or make it yourself. If you're picking a financially arranged item, be aware of included sugar.

Outline

Kefir is an aged dairy drink with numerous medical advantages identified with its probiotic content. Although by and large produced using bovine's milk, kefir is additionally accessible in non-dairy structures.

8. Garlic

Garlic is a plant nourishment that is firmly identified with onions, leeks and shallots. It's a decent wellspring of manganese, nutrient C, nutrient B6, selenium and fiber.

Garlic is a mainstream culinary fixing because of its unmistakable flavor; however, it has likewise been utilized for its therapeutic advantages for a considerable length of time.

Research shows that garlic might be powerful in diminishing cholesterol and circulatory strain, just as supporting invulnerable capacity.

In addition, sulfur-containing mixes in garlic may even assume a job in forestalling specific sorts of malignant growth.

Outline

Garlic is a supplement rich nourishment utilized for its restorative advantages for a considerable length of time. It might be helpful for supporting invulnerable capacity and lessening your danger of coronary illness and certain tumors.

9. Olive Oil

Olive oil is a characteristic oil extricated from the product of olive trees and one of the pillars of the Mediterranean diet.

It's greatest cases to wellbeing are its significant levels of monounsaturated unsaturated fats (MUFAs) and polyphenolic mixes.

Adding olive oil to your diet may diminish irritation and your danger of specific ailments, for example, coronary illness and diabetes.

It additionally contains cancer prevention agents, for example, nutrients E and K, which can shield against cell harm from oxidative pressure.

Outline

Olive oil is one of the standard fat sources in the Mediterranean diet. It might be valuable in lessening coronary illness, diabetes and other provocative conditions.

10. Ginger

Ginger originates from the foundation of a blossoming plant from China. It's utilized as both a culinary flavor enhancer and for its numerous restorative impacts.

Ginger root contains cell reinforcements, for example, gingerol, that might be answerable for huge numbers of the announced medical advantages related with this nourishment.

Ginger might be successful for overseeing queasiness and lessening torment from intense and constant fiery conditions.

It might likewise lessen your danger of constant sicknesses, for example, coronary illness, dementia and certain malignant growths.

Ginger is accessible crisp, as an oil or squeeze and in dried/powdered structures. It's anything but difficult to fuse into soups, sautés, sauces and teas.

Outline

Ginger is utilized for its flavor and potential restorative impacts. It might be valuable in treating sickness, torment and forestalling certain interminable illnesses.

11. Turmeric (Curcumin)

Turmeric is a brilliant yellow flavor that is firmly identified with ginger. Initially from India, it's utilized for cooking and its restorative advantages.

Curcumin is the dynamic compound in turmeric. It has intense cancer prevention agent and mitigating impacts and is the focal point of most research encompassing turmeric.

Studies show that curcumin might be powerful in treating and forestalling constant infections, for example, malignancy, coronary illness and diabetes.

It might likewise help wound mending and agony decrease.

One downside of utilizing curcumin restoratively is that it's not effectively consumed by your body, yet its ingestion can be improved by matching it with fats or different flavors, for example, dark pepper.

Outline

The dynamic compound in turmeric, curcumin, is related with a few restorative impacts. Curcumin isn't effectively retained and ought to be combined with substances that upgrade its assimilation, for example, dark pepper.

12. Salmon

Salmon is a profoundly nutritious fish stuffed with sound fats, protein, B nutrients, potassium and selenium.

It's probably the best wellspring of omega-3 unsaturated fats, which are known for an assortment of medical advantages, for example, diminishing irritation.

Remembering salmon for your diet may likewise bring down your danger of coronary illness and diabetes and assist you with keeping up a sound weight.

A potential disadvantage of eating salmon and different kinds of fish is their conceivable tainting with substantial metals and other natural poisons.

You can stay away from potential negative impacts by restricting your utilization of fish to a few servings for every week (41).

Synopsis

Salmon is a decent wellspring of numerous supplements, particularly omega-3 unsaturated fats. Point of confinement your utilization of salmon to keep away from potential negative impacts from contaminants basic in fish and fish.

13. Avocado

Avocado is an exceptionally nutritious natural product; however, it's often treated progressively like a vegetable in culinary applications.

It's plentiful in numerous supplements, including fiber, nutrients, minerals and sound fats.

Like olive oil, avocado is high in monounsaturated fats (MUFAs). Oleic corrosive is the most transcendent MUFA in avocado, which is connected to diminished irritation in the body.

Eating avocado may decrease your danger of coronary illness, diabetes, metabolic disorder and specific kinds of malignant growth.

Outline

Avocados are supplement rich, high-fiber natural products that may assume a job in diminishing irritation and ceaseless infections.

14. Sweet Potato

The sweet potato is a root vegetable stacked with numerous supplements, including potassium, fiber and nutrients An and C.

They're additionally a decent wellspring of carotenoids, a sort of cell reinforcement that may lessen your danger of specific kinds of malignant growth.

In spite of their sweet flavor, sweet potatoes don't build glucose as much as you would anticipate. Curiously, they may really improve glucose control in those with type 2 diabetes.

Outline

Sweet potatoes are a profoundly nutritious nourishment stacked with carotenoids, which have solid cell reinforcement properties. They may likewise be advantageous for glucose control.

15. Mushrooms

The absolute most regular assortments of eatable mushrooms are button, portobello, shiitake, crimini and clam mushrooms.

Despite the fact that supplement content changes relying upon the sort, mushrooms contain nutrient A, potassium, fiber, and a few cell reinforcements not present in most different nourishments.

Strikingly, eating more mushrooms is related with more noteworthy utilization of vegetables all in all, adding to a general progressively nutritious diet.

Because of their one of a kind cell reinforcement content, mushrooms may likewise assume a job in lessening irritation and forestalling specific sorts of malignancies.

Another super element of mushrooms is that rural waste items are utilized to develop them. This makes mushrooms a supportable part of a sound nourishment framework.

Outline

Mushrooms are loaded with supplements and may decrease your danger of specific ailments. Furthermore, mushrooms are a manageable nourishment decision.

16. Kelp

Kelp is a term used to portray certain supplement rich ocean vegetables. It's most normally devoured in Asian food however is picking up notoriety in different pieces of the world because of its healthy benefit.

Ocean growth packs numerous supplements, including nutrient K, folate, iodine and fiber.

These sea vegetables are a wellspring of novel bioactive mixes — not ordinarily show in land-vegetables — which may have cell reinforcement impacts.

A portion of these mixes may likewise diminish your danger of malignant growth, coronary illness, heftiness and diabetes.

Synopsis

Ocean growth is a gathering of exceptionally nutritious ocean vegetables that may assume a job in ensuring against certain interminable illnesses.

17. Watermelon

Low in sugar and high in nutrients An and C, this midyear treat is the ideal, amazing failure calorie nibble. Studies recommend watermelon could likewise possibly bring down circulatory strain and diminish the danger of cardiovascular sickness. Furthermore, the lycopene in watermelon could help shield the body from UV beams and malignant growth.

18. Apples

Say it with us, individuals: "Fiber is acceptable." And apples are an incredible low-calorie source. (A medium-sized apple tips the scales at under 100 calories.) Plus, increasing apple consumption has been related with decreased danger of cardiovascular sickness, certain malignant growths, diabetes, and asthma.

SIRTFOOD RECIPE

Superfoods are probably the most healthfully thick nourishments on earth. While a considerable lot of us are simply getting on to the superfood pattern, many have been utilized for a huge number of years by indigenous individuals as different types of common prescription. These force stuffed nourishments arrive in an assortment of structures from seeds, berries, gels and powders, each accompanying a different advantage.

1. Orange, Fig and Baobab Cheesecake

Recall the baobab tree from "The Little Prince?" Who might have believed that baobab was a superfood in addition to it tastes extraordinary! This Orange, Fig and Baobab Cheesecake is a tasty, velvety treat that is made altogether of common entire nourishments so you can appreciate each significant piece!

2. Goji Berry and Hazelnut Cacao Truffles

Goji berries are little yet enthusiastic about nourishment. These Goji Berry and Hazelnut Cacao Truffles are abounded in squashed goji berries. They're brisk and simple, crude, veggie lovr, sans gluten, without dairy, paleo-accommodating, no-heat, and no have no refined sugar. Gracious definitely, they're extremely scrumptious as well!

3. Mint Matcha Chip Ice Cream

This Mint Matcha Chocolate Chip Ice Cream is smooth, liberal and bravo! It has matcha green tea in it which gives it shading as well as it's a superfood. In addition to the fact that this is anything but difficult to make thus reviving, it'll immediately turn into your new most loved flavor!

4. Bubbly Coconut, Lime and Mint Kombucha Elixir

This Fizzy Coconut, Lime and Mint Kombucha Elixir is reviving, tastes astonishing, looks beautiful, is hydrating, feeding and loaded with solid probiotics! Both coconut and fermented tea are considered superfoods. Check out it at home and intrigue companions with this pretty mocktail.

5. Crude Chocolate Mint Grasshopper Pie

This Raw Chocolate Mint Grasshopper Pie is a genuine group pleaser and ideal for an uncommon event with loved ones. Where's the superfood? Spirulina, a sort of green growth, gives this pie its beautiful shading and huge amounts of solid supplements.

6. Rainbow Vegetable Saffron Millet Croquettes

Antiquated grains are superfoods and it's enjoyable to attempt new ones you may not be comfortable with like millet. These Rainbow Vegetable Saffron Millet Croquettes are an incredible method to attempt it. The outside gets fresh and within remains delicate. You'll begin to look all starry eyed at this grain and this dish.

7. Kimchi Kale Salad

Aged nourishments are superfoods and an extraordinary method to get probiotics into your diet. Eating kimchi, a Korean dish like sauerkraut, is a heavenly method to do it. Kimchi includes such a lot of flavor, surface, and shading to nourishment. The crunch and harshness are particularly brilliant right now Salad made with avocado, kneaded kale, chickpeas, and broiled sweet potatoes – which all happen to be superfoods too.

8. Hand crafted Dark Chocolate Chunks

Genuine chocolate – the sort accepted to hold enchanted, or even celestial, properties. All things considered, we have been hearing that a tad of dim chocolate is useful for the heart and certainly for the spirit. This Homemade Dark Chocolate Chunks formula lets you control the measure of sweetness and salt in your chocolate. That is the excellence of making your own.

9. Broiled Cauliflower and Avocado Cream Pitas

Cauliflower and avocado are both dietary powerhouses and these Roasted Cauliflower and Avocado Cream Pitas are the tastiest approach to practice good eating habits. The spiced broiled cauliflower and avocado cream are an agreeable flavor blend that preferences great on totally anything.

10. Best Ever Forbidden Rice Salad

Dark rice is a superfood and the way that it's called prohibited rice just makes it much progressively captivating. This Forbidden Rice Salad is simple, fast, and ensured to intrigue. Dark rice has a simmered nutty flavor and matches well with a wide range of veggies and greens. The ginger miso dressing goes splendidly with the sweet potatoes and nutty rice.

11. Zesty Kale and Quinoa Black Bean Salad

Kale and quinoa are both superfoods. When you set up them with solid dark beans right now and Quinoa Black Bean Salad, you have a wholesome trifecta! Dark colored rice, dark beans, peppers, corn, salsa, lettuce, guacamole – what's not to adore?

12. Chia Pudding with Blueberries

Chia seeds are sound and berries are additionally superfoods. This Chia Pudding with Blueberries is smooth, sweet and sustaining. This treat is so liberal and delectable, you'll overlook it's beneficial for you.

13. Plantain Sweet Potato Tacos with Guacamole

These Plantain Sweet Potato Tacos with Guacamole are actually as they sound – loaded down with plantains, sweet potatoes and dark beans and bested with a basic guacamole. They're veggie lover, sans gluten and a phenomenal lunch or supper alternative!

14. Chocolate Einkorn Cake

Is it cake? Is it a brownie? Whatever you call it, this Chocolate Einkorn Cake is delightful. It's a super chocolatey, not excessively sweet, wet cake-brownie bar ... and it's incredible. Einkorn wheat is old wheat that has never been hereditarily modified so it's solid and simpler to process.

15. Coconut Flour Porridge with Roasted Apricots

Did you realize that coconut flour makes a thick and delightful gluten and without grain porridge? Disregard your common cereal and attempt this yummy, simple breakfast of Coconut Flour Porridge! It's particularly delicious when topped with sweet caramelized apricots, however mess around with your own preferred garnishes.

16. Sound Hearty Whole Wheat Pancakes with Flax

It's constantly enjoyable to add foods grown from the ground to the hitter yet in some cases you need a flapjack formula that is somewhat more unbiased in enhance. A formula that asks for sweet fixings and a streaming waterway of maple syrup. However, obviously, it despite everything must be sound. These Healthy Hearty Whole Wheat Pancakes fit the bill impeccably. They top you off with Omega rich flax all while as yet tasting flavorful close by some new leafy foods mug of espresso or tea.

17. Spring Onion Farro Fritters with Fresh Peas, Asparagus, Radish and Tahini Mint Dressing

If farro is another grain for you, these Spring Onion Farro Fritters with Fresh Peas, Asparagus and Radishes are an extraordinary method to get presented. They are entire nourishments, plant-based thus scrumptious. Present with the mint tahini dressing which is tasty and furthermore solid.

18. Bahn Mi Salad with Pickled Vegetables and Vietnamese Croutons

Cured nourishments are superfoods and this Banh Mi Salad with Pickled Vegetables is a super dish. It's loaded up with dynamic flavors and the Vietnamese bread garnishes on top include crunch. This formula serves two huge plates of mixed greens and is veggie lover, protein-pressed and without nut with a sans gluten alternative accessible.

19. Crude Apple Pie with Goji Berries and Nutmeg

You might be thinking about how crusty fruit-filled treat can be a superfood? When it's this Raw Apple Pie with Goji Berries and Nutmeg, it can. It has sound apples, superfood goji berries and it's crude so there's no batter. It is as nutritious as it is delectable! It is additionally exquisite topped with coconut yogurt.

20. Avocado and Veggie Spring Rolls

Avocados are superfoods and we are so cheerful about that. These Avocado and Veggie Spring Rolls are so flavorful. Loaded up with crunchy veggies and velvety avocado with bunches of Asian flavors, we prescribe making a great deal because these will vanish before your eyes.

21. Broccoli and Coconut Soup

This Broccoli and Coconut Soup is a lively, delightful and exceptionally nutritious mix of broccoli, spinach, lemon, ginger, and coconut milk that will warm you and feed you through the cooler winter months or just whenever you have to heat up inside.

22. Wild Rice Salad with Orange, Sweet Potato, Cherries and Pecans

This Wild Rice Salad is so pretty thus bravo. It's overflowing with a wide range of superfoods. Zest up your typical plate of mixed greens life with this delicious mix of wild rice, sweet potato, orange, fruits, and walnuts. It's the best of fall in a bowl!

23. Dark Bean Hemp Burgers

These Black Bean Hemp Burgers are so ideal for lunch, supper, nibble, even breakfast. They're likewise an ideal travel partner that will get together effectively and keep you full for a considerable length of time, on account of all the protein, fiber, and supplements.

24. Fig Hazelnut Rosemary Granola with Fig Breakfast 'Decent' Cream

Dried figs are superfoods and they're doubly solid right now Rosemary Granola with Fig Breakfast 'Decent' Cream since they are utilized twice! This yummy breakfast combo has dried figs that make the granola magnificently chewy and solidified green figs zoomed up until cushy in the "pleasant" cream.

25. Green Bean and Wild Rice Salad

When served warm, this Green Bean and Wild Rice Salad is sufficiently healthy to eat during even the coldest winter months and it has a few superfoods in it. Crunchy almonds, chewy cranberries and sun-dried tomatoes, tart olives, and generous wild rice give an intriguing blend of surfaces that will make them desire more!

SCIENCE BEHIND SIRTFOODS

Hardly any things are so profoundly contaminated by trends, cheats and misrepresentation as nourishment. All things considered, it is through a perspective of sound wariness that we should see any new diet. The most recent to stand out as truly newsworthy is the Sirtfood diet which, if we are to fully trust claims, will help with weight loss just as offering different advantages, for example, "invigorating restoration and cell fix".

For the unenlightened, this most recent diet is based around utilization of nourishments which may associate with a group of proteins known as sirtuin proteins, or SIRT1 - SIRT7. Adding to the diet's undoubted request is the way that the best sources as far as anyone knows incorporate red wine and chocolate, just as citrus organic products, blueberries and kale. During the initial three days, calorie admission is restricted (1,000 calories for every day) and comprises of three Sirtfood green juices, in addition to a typical feast rich in "Sirtfoods". On days four to seven, calorie admission is expanded (1,500 calories) and comprises of two juices and two dinners. Past that the suggestion is to eat a reasonable diet rich in sirtuin nourishments, alongside further green juices. Prawns and salmon additionally include in the supper plans.

It sounds scrumptious – and sirtuins are for sure embroiled in a wide scope of cell forms including digestion, maturing and circadian musicality. The diet is additionally situated to a limited extent, on calorie limitation. The nutritionists behind this recommend the diet "impacts the body's capacity to consume fat and lifts the metabolic framework".

The diet decoded

So, what do we think about this diet? From a scientific viewpoint, the appropriate response is practically nothing. Sirtuins add to guideline of fat and glucose digestion considering changes in vitality levels. They may likewise have an impact in the impact of calorie limitation on upgrades in maturing. This is maybe by means of sirtuins' consequences for high-impact (or mitochondrial) digestion, bringing down of responsive oxygen species (free radicals) and increments in cancer prevention agent proteins.

Besides, explore recommends that transgenic mice with more elevated levels of SIRT6 live significantly longer than wild-type mice, and that changes in SIRT6 articulation might be important in maturing of some human skin cells. SIRT2 likewise has been shown to moderate metazoan (yeast) maturing.

It sounds noteworthy and the diet makes them gleam surveys, however, none of this speaks to convincing scientific proof of the Sirtfood Diet effects affecting genuine individuals. It would be a colossal over-extrapolation to expect that lab look into directed on mice, yeast and human undifferentiated organisms has any bearing on certifiable wellbeing results – polluted as they are by a huge number of perplexing factors.

The study of weight loss

Surely the diet will seem to work for certain individuals. Be that as it may, scientific evidence of any diet's triumphs is an altogether different issue. Obviously, the perfect investigation to think about the adequacy of a diet on weight loss (or some other result, for example, maturing) would require an adequately huge example – agent of the populace we are keen on – and arbitrary allotment to a treatment or control gathering. Results would then be checked over a satisfactory timeframe with severe command over perplexing factors, for example, different practices that may emphatically or contrarily influence the results of enthusiasm (smoking, for example, or work out).

This exploration would be constrained by techniques, for example, self-detailing and memory, yet would go some approach to finding the viability of this diet. Research of this nature, be that as it may, doesn't exist and we ought to therefore be careful when deciphering fundamental science – all things considered, human cells in a tissue culture dish likely respond differently to the phones in a living individual.

Further uncertainty is thrown over this diet when we think about a portion of the specific cases. Losses of seven pounds in a single week are unreasonable and are probably not going to reflect changes to muscle versus fat. For the initial three days, dieters expend around 1000 kcal every day – around 40–half of what the vast majority require. This will bring about a quick loss of glycogen (a put away type of sugar) from skeletal muscle and the liver.

In any case, for each gram of put away glycogen we likewise store around 2.7 grams of water, and water is overwhelming. So, for all the lost glycogen, we additionally lose going with water – and thus weight. Also, diets that are too prohibitive are extremely difficult to follow and bring about increments in hunger invigorating hormones, for example, ghrelin. Weight (glycogen and water) will therefore come back to ordinary if the desire to eat wins out.

When all is said in done, utilization of the scientific strategy to the investigation of nourishment is difficult. It is often impractical to complete fake treatment controlled preliminaries with any level of natural legitimacy, and the wellbeing results that we are often keen on happen over numerous years, making research configuration testing. Besides, contemplates in enormous populaces rely upon shockingly shortsighted and innocent information assortment techniques, for example, memory and self-detailing, which produce famously questionable information. Against this foundation commotion, nourishment look into has a difficult activity.

Is there a convenient solution?

Sadly, not. Sensationalized features and often hyperbolic portrayal of scientific information brings about the apparently unlimited contentions about what – and how much – we ought to eat, further fueling our fixation on a "handy solution" or wonder fix, which is an endemic social issue.

For the reasons sketched out, the Sirtfood diet ought to be relegated to the prevailing fashion heap – in any event from a scientific point of view. Considering the proof, we have, to propose in any case is, best case scenario false and even under the least favorable conditions deluding and harming to the real points of general wellbeing procedure. The diet is probably not going to offer any profit to populaces confronting a plague of diabetes, prowling in the shadow of weight. As expressed obviously by others, exceptional diets don't work and dieting all in all is anything but a general wellbeing answer for social orders where the greater part of grown-ups are overweight.

By and by, the best system is long haul conduct change joined with political and ecological impact, focused on expanded physical movement and some type of cognizant authority over what we eat. It is anything but a convenient solution, yet it will work.

There's another big name diet on the square, and it's sponsored by none other than Adele. The British vocalist lyricist's emotional change and right around 50-pound weight loss got everybody discussing the Sirtfood Diet – which includes initiating your 'thin quality' by remembering certain nourishments for your diet. Chocolate, red wine and espresso are not beyond reach and you can lose as much as seven pounds every week.

Like most prevailing fashion diets, it sounds excessively great to be valid, or possibly, feasible. In this way, here's a more intensive look.

What goes into it?

The term 'sirt nourishments' was promoted not long ago by British nutritionists Aidan Goggins and Glen Matten with the arrival of their book, The Sirtfood Diet. It advocates a diet wealthy in nourishments that invigorate sirtuin, a specific protein accepted to advance weight loss through accelerating digestion and expanding strong proficiency. Sirtuins are additionally connected with life span since it forestalls aggravation and advances cell development.

The diet itself is comprised of two phases. During the initial three days of stage one, calorie admission is restricted to 1000 cals a day spread across three sirtfood green juices and one standard feast with sirtuin-rich nourishments. In days 4–7, 1500 calories are devoured through two juices and two standard suppers daily. In arrange two, which endures 14 days, dieters eat three adjusted sirtfood-rich suppers alongside one serving of green juice. Post that, the proposal is to eat a fair diet rich in sirtuin nourishments and green juices. The creators demand that the Sirtfood Diet centers around eating the nourishments you love and not removing food sources or slandering entire nutritional categories.

Sirtuin-rich nourishments

Fortunately, the sirtuin-rich nourishments suggested by the book are all around nutritious and useful for a great many people. These incorporate pecans, strawberries, espresso, kale, celery with leaves, additional virgin olive oil, buckwheat, stew, cocoa (in any event 85-percent unadulterated), matcha, green tea, medjool dates, red chicory, red onion, red wine, arugula, soy and turmeric. The green juice contains Kale, parsley, rocket, celery, apple, lemon and matcha.

GREENS

Does it work?

Any diet that confines your calorie-admission is probably going to work at the outset and individuals have detailed dropping numbers on the scale. Be that as it may, is this weight loss practical? "Regarding weight loss and boosting digestion, individuals may have encountered a seven pound weight loss on the scales, yet as far as I can tell this will be liquid. Consuming and losing fat requires significant investment so it is amazingly far-fetched this weight loss is a loss of fat," dietitian Emer Delaney clarifies in BBC GoodFood.

The genuine test lies in guaranteeing that the weight remains off and your body gets all its basic supplements simultaneously. While there's no denying that the sirtfoods prescribed are in fact sound, there's constantly a peril of overabundance. A lot of cocoa, wine or olive oil will include calories regardless. Also, calorie necessities rely upon your tallness, sexual orientation and action levels, so there's actually nobody size-fit-all diet

Discontinuous fasting (IF) has huge amounts of advantages, including weight loss, forestalling diabetes, and lessening your danger of disease. Numerous individuals who follow IF state that it's helped them appreciate their dinners more and comprehend the difference among appetite and desires. It has likewise helped them get through weight loss levels.

"IF causes you to feel great since you're disposing of the aggravation," says, Wendy Scinta, M.D., leader of the Obesity Medicine Association and an individual from Prevention's Medical Review Board. "I follow the 16:8 diet and find that when I endorse IF to patients who need to shed 100 pounds and can't lose the last 15 pounds, IF causes them arrive."

In any case, IF isn't for everybody (Dr. Scinta doesn't suggest it for individuals who have a background marked by scattered eating or pregnant ladies), and it's essential to comprehend the symptoms that accompany it.

Regardless of what sort of irregular fasting technique you're keen on following, here are symptoms you should know.

1. Beginners may feel hypoglycemic.

From the outset, you may encounter hypoglycemia, a condition brought about by extremely low glucose levels. This can prompt migraines, expanded pulse, dazedness, and queasiness, according to Dr. Scinta. Goodness, and awful dispositions—nobody's cheerful when they're confining nourishment. "When you don't eat, your body will initially consume the glycogen (put away glucose) in your liver and muscles (subsequently feeling aggravated from the start), then it will start to consume fat for fuel," says Frances Largeman-Roth, R.D.N., nourishment and wellbeing master, creator of Eating in Color and maker of the FLR VIP program, says. In any case, as your body turns out to be more keto versatile and figures out how to run on fat rather than glucose, Dr. Scinta says hypoglycemia turns out to be to a lesser extent a worry.

In any case, if you keep on feeling woozy or bleary eyed after some time, Largeman-Roth says to eat something—regardless of whether it's a little bite. "Shedding pounds is never an adequate motivation to drop," she says.

What's more, make a point to fuel up on solid, fulfilling nourishments during suppers. Slender protein, leafy foods, entire grains, and sound fats, for example, avocados, nuts, and extra-virgin olive oil will keep your glucose levels adjusted during your quick and give the supplements your body needs to work appropriately.

Dr. Scinta says she often finds that individuals on IF battle to get enough protein, so make sure to eat routinely, including tidbits, when you're not fasting. "You should plan to get at any rate one gram of protein for each kilogram of weight every day," she says.

2. You'll hunger for carbs and prepared nourishments less.

Dr. Scinta says that numerous individuals who follow IF make some better memories at keeping their glucose levels adjusted. In such a case that powers you to quit eating at a specific time, you'll fuel up on all the more fulfilling nourishments, similar to lean protein and fiber, to remain full during your quick. "What I've found with IF is that it's helped me watch my carb consumption," Dr. Scinta says. "You're eating to such an extent; however, you're not eating as a significant part of the terrible stuff."

IF additionally advances satiety through the creation of craving decreasing hormones. A recent report from Obesity recommends that IF can help decline ghrelin levels—the hormone that animates hunger—in overweight grown-ups and improve individuals' capacity to switch between consuming carbs for vitality and consuming fat for vitality.

"There are people who eat around evening time because of fatigue or stress, not on the grounds that they're really ravenous. Putting guardrails on the occasions they can eat may assist them with abstaining from eating when they don't should be," Largeman-Roth says.

Dr. Scinta and Largeman-Roth additionally encourage individuals to remain hydrated while fasting since individuals will in general mistake hunger for hunger.

"When individuals quick in the first part of the day, they drink a great deal of espresso, which is a diuretic, and neglect to drink water," Dr. Scinta says. "Each capacity in the body requires water, so remaining hydrated is unfathomably significant," Largeman-Roth says. "We get about 20% of our water consumption from the nourishment we eat, so when we quick, we're losing a significant wellspring of hydration," she says.

3. You'll improve your insulin affectability.

A recent report in Cell Metabolism found that men with prediabetes who followed IF improved their insulin affectability, despite the fact that they didn't get thinner. How can it work, precisely? Whenever you eat, your body discharges the hormone insulin to move sugar from your circulatory system into your cells for vitality. Be that as it may, individuals with prediabetes don't react well to insulin so their glucose levels remain raised. Expanding the time between suppers can help on the grounds that your body discharges less insulin.

In any case, Dr. Scinta says that individuals who are on insulin-subordinate drugs ought to counsel with their primary care physician before following IF in light of the fact that it can influence the adequacy of their treatment. "Individuals with type 1 or 2 diabetes are on these meds to bring down their glucose, so they have to have steady dinners to forestall spikes in their glucose," Dr. Scinta says.

4. Your workouts may endure a shot.

Following IF and working out is absolutely protected, however you'll have to make a few acclimations to your timetable with the goal that you're not running on void. Let's assume you're following the 5:2 diet: Doing low-affect workouts rather than progressively serious ones, like weightlifting, running, and HIIT, on days when you're constraining calories can enable your body to change in accordance with the new requests. As your body becomes acclimated to consuming fat for fuel, the power of your workouts won't be as a lot of a worry.

So, the exact opposite thing you need to do is drop during your HIIT class, so Dr. Scinta prescribes timing your workouts toward the start or end of your quick. Along these lines, you can appreciate a pre-or post-workout nibble. Nourishments that are anything but difficult to process, like a smoothie, low-fat yogurt, and nutty spread with toast work better pre-workout, while nourishments with a higher carb-to-protein proportion, for example, a bowl of cereal, are perfect for post-workout.

Researchers drove by Dr Naiara Beraza at the Institute of Food Research on the Norwich Research Park are exploring the systems supporting the alleged useful impacts of the 'Sirtfood Diet'.

Sirtfoods burst onto the wellbeing and sustenance scene prior this year, making a sprinkle in the media, with a few prominent competitors including Olympic gold-medallist Sir Ben Ainslie changing over their dietary propensities according to The Independent.

While this news may urge potential dieters to head out close by such brandishing VIPs, analysts at the IFR are provisional and propose unquestionably more research is required into the scientific premise behind the physiological advantages that the nourishments included are intended to convey.

So, what is the scientific proof behind these cases?

A large number of these nourishments may to be sure have medical advantages for us when we eat them. There is acceptable proof that individuals who have diets high in vegetables and organic products have a decreased danger of creating ceaseless conditions. A portion of these nourishments contain bioactives, which are natural particles that impact living cells, and that may likewise show medical advantages. IFR has a program of research taking a gander at bioactive, to attempt to locate the best proof for how they are processed and the components by which they may profit wellbeing.

There are a wide range of manners by which these advantages might be deciphered. Defenders of the SIRTFOOD diet guarantee that bioactive mixes initiate proteins called sirtuins. These sirtuins trigger the statement of qualities that they connect to cell restoration and fix, concealment of craving and weight loss. Nourishments rich in these bioactives have been marked 'sirtfoods'; predominantly products of the soil including blueberries, rocket, celery, kale and apples and other nourishment types, for example, 85% dim chocolate and red wine. In any case, the proof connecting these sirtfoods back to human medical advantages, by means of enactment of sirtuins, is as yet uncertain.

We realize that there are seven sirtuins in our body yet we don't have the foggiest idea what they all do. The most notable is sirtuin

1. There is proof from tests in mice that overexpressing SIRT1 gives sound maturing and that these mice are ensured against high fat diet-actuated metabolic disorder, described by corpulence and greasy liver. Resveratrol, a proposed SIRT bioactive found in the skin of red grapes, has been appeared to actuate the SIRT1 quality, dragging out the lifespan of lower living beings yet not warm blooded creatures. Flavonoids found in chocolate are likewise known to initiate SIRT1 in worms.

Dr Beraza proposes that the scientific premise utilized for advancement of this diet is doubtlessly founded on the effect of resveratrol expanding the lifespan of lower creatures, for example, sprouting yeast. The cell components by which resveratrol acts stays dubious and starting at 2016, the medical advantages in people presently can't seem to be demonstrated indisputably.

Another significant point is that the measure of bioactive found in these nourishments might be not even close to enough to have any advantageous impacts. While it's demonstrated that certain bioactives can actuate SIRT1, we don't know whether the levels in nourishments in amounts that individuals normally eat can encourage this enactment. Different components to consider are that eating these nourishments may infer a decrease in calorie admission, as the greater part of the related nourishments will in general be lower in sugars and fats, with diminished calorie utilization known to actuate SIRT1. Exercise may likewise be expanded in people participating in such a diet as most diets prescribe expanded exercise. Exercise is known to incite SIRT1 action so the nourishment itself may not assume such a significant job.

So, what move would it be advisable for us to make to additionally examine SIRT1?

Dr. Bereza proposes that we should attempt to characterize the instruments basic any helpful impacts and how SIRT1 overexpression ensures against a high fat diet. There might be specific conditions where a lot of SIRT1 movement could prompt unintended impacts. Late research indicated that SIRT1 overexpression in mice delivered hindered liver recovery and a few different papers by different research bunches have demonstrated that SIRT1 is exceptionally communicated in liver tumor tests. Sirtuin 1 is an amazing particle that controls basic metabolic pathways, cell assurance frameworks and manages provocative reaction so it is important to characterize in which organs SIRT1 has impacts, and what those impacts are.

While some work has been done on the liver with respect to these systems, there is a nonattendance of research which endeavors to characterize the job of SIRT1 in the liver-gut hub. Her group at the IFR will examine this job to show whether SIRT1 actuation must be organ specific to harvest the advantageous impacts with the goal that we may reason the best technique to deliver viable SIRT1-based medications.

So, should perusers forsake the SIRT send?

"I think not" affirms Dr. Beraza "However simply because huge numbers of the 'Sirtfoods' can be incorporated as a major aspect of a sound lifestyle which are known to present other dietary advantages. Dieters would likewise be better encouraged to consolidate these nourishments, as a blend of the mixes will probably have more prominent favorable circumstances than eating one nourishment type alone. Pathways other than SIRT1 can be actuated, upgrading the helpful impacts while likewise making dinners less exhausting! It is additionally essential to join these nourishments with non-SIRT nourishments as a feature of a fair diet including protein and suggested levels of fat nearby customary exercise."

In general, the SIRT1 message is idealistic with regards to stoutness, high fat diets and metabolic disorder, yet so as to expand the potential that these bioactives may have, we should completely examine the instruments behind these impacts, with specific accentuation on the job of SIRT in the liver-gut pivot. While an 'enchantment pill' to fix weight may at present be distant, work at the IFR could reveal more insight into the mind boggling systems embroiled in SIRT1 articulation to all the more likely comprehend a conceivably helpful dietary road.

CONCLUSION

'We don't yet have the proof that specific nourishments actuate this more than others – or to which specific tissues they'd be gainful,' says. 'Regardless of whether sirtfoods do trigger weight loss, the sheer amount we'd have to eat might be unmanageable.' He focuses to resveratrol, the polyphenol in red wine and the most notable of all sirtuin activators.

Resveratrol shot to popularity in 2003 when a research facility of researchers run by David Sinclair found that this compound, found most normally in the skins of red grapes, copied the impacts of calorie limitation and actuated sirtuins that drawn out the life of cells. Subsequently the 'red wine encourages you live more' way of thinking that is become progressively mainstream bandied about at the bar.

Be that as it may, Hirschey brings up, 'most of studies have been done utilizing test frameworks in the lab, generally on mice or natural product flies, or legitimately into cells. To get resveratrol's enemy of maturing impacts from red wine, you'd need to drink up to 40 liters every day.' Which makes you wonder how much kale you'd should pack so as to get thinner.

The nutraceutical business is as of now one stage ahead, with resveratrol supplements effectively accessible. Be watchful, in any case, of simply popping some sirt-enacting pills or binding your smoothies with resveratrol powder, as one examination from the University of Copenhagen has demonstrated that expanded supplementation of the cancer prevention agent neutralized the great impacts of activity.

Actually, you don't need to, particularly not to begin. Currently, we are adapted to be snappy and proficient, and to be brisk we have been acquainted with inexpensive food and handled nourishment.

I think what many individuals foul up as do I (during the time spent fixing my diet) is to think about the nourishment being removed, so obviously with that sort of reasoning it turns out to be almost difficult to go for a superfood/rawfood diet. Be that as it may, if we have a go at including the superfood/rawfood into our current diet, things like crude vegetables, sprouts, natural products, and juices, you won't experience considerable difficulties exchanging. In the wake of adding these natural products to your diet you may not be as eager and when you're not ravenous, you won't surrender to purchasing inexpensive food and prepared nourishment.

Since you will have more opportunity to consider your buys and you have gotten increasingly acclimated with eating more advantageous. If you need that steak or even a McDonald's cheeseburger, you can get yourself it, and it will taste so much better... or on the other hand you might be fortunate to the point that you won't need it by any stretch of the imagination. When you begin eating Superfoods however, you will begin to see how great you feel and the amount more vitality you have, that cheeseburger just won't look as great to you any longer.

During the time spent changing your diet and after changing you would like no doubt however, that you're getting enough of the correct sorts of sustenance. Eating Superfoods/crude nourishments isn't simply enough you have to do some exploration on the most proficient method to add your fundamental proteins to your new diet. Recall before you got your protein through your meat yet now you need to get it through your vegetables and crude nourishment, so you have to recognize what to eat and what blends you have to eat to get enough proteins.

One approach to do this is to present another vegetable or crude dish each week. If you are to purchase another vegetable every week and become acclimated to the taste by utilizing it in your feast the entire week. By doing this you will adjust to the new tastes and surfaces and you will begin feeling more regrettable and more terrible for each time you go for inexpensive food or handled nourishment.

CPSIA information can be obtained
at www.ICGtesting.com
Printed in the USA
LVHW010531110121
676184LV00007B/252